LABORATORY
RELATED
MEASURES OF
PATIENT
OUTCOMES

LABORATORY-RELATED MEASURES OF PATIENT OUTCOMES:
An Introduction

Edited by

Michael G. Bissell, MD, PhD, MPH

Professor of Pathology MCP/Hahnemann University School of Medicine and
Director of Clinical Pathology
Allegheny General Hospital
Pittsburgh, Pennsylvania

AACC Press
2101 L Street, NW, Suite 202
Washington, DC 20037-1526

1 2 3 4 5 6 7 8 9 0   I C P   02 01 00

Library of Congress Cataloging-in-Publication Data

Laboratory-related measures of patient outcomes : an introduction / edited by
    Michael G. Bissell.
            p. ; cm.
Includes bibliographical references and index.
ISBN 1-890883-26-3 (alk. Paper)
1. Outcome assessment (Medical care) 2. Medical protocol. I. Bissell,   Michael G.
[DNLM: 1. Laboratory Techniques and Procedures.   2. Research—methods. 3.
Diagnostic Tests, Routine. 4. Outcome Assessment (Health Care). QY 20 L123 2000]
R853.O87 L33 2000
616.07'56—dc21   99-059233

Contents

SECTION III: PRACTICAL APPLICATIONS

Preface

The field of laboratory-related outcomes research is in its infancy. Only a handful of really useful studies have been produced in this very difficult-to-study area. Yet the need for the development of the field is rapidly becoming unquestioned.

Managed care organizations and health-care policymakers are long since used to having valid information about the relative cost-effectiveness and cost-benefit of drugs and other therapies, but there is, as yet, no comparable body of information regarding in vitro diagnostic testing. Recent estimates have appeared in the medical literature that as much as 50–60% of all clinical laboratory testing may be unnecessary. Within health plans, quality managers responsible for the creation of practice guidelines have a real need to know of the valid bases that may exist for determining the true value of laboratory testing in the clinical context. This can best be done via outcomes research, and thus an understanding of the specific issues peculiar to determining the impact of diagnostics on patient outcomes is key.

The in vitro diagnostic (IVD) industry has a vital survival interest in the establishment of agreed-upon methodologies for the conduct of laboratory-related outcomes studies. Their ability to establish the value of their products, and thus their place in the market, is becoming steadily more dependent upon an evidence-based approach. Clinical pathologists have never been more sincere or highly motivated to seek ways to genuinely add value to the health-care system than they are today. Becoming involved more directly with patient care and with managing the health of populations is being increasingly recognized as the pathologist's future role. Laboratory-related outcomes work will form the scientific basis of this prospect. If laboratory managers and directors are to become more involved with clinical process management in their institutions, and are to broaden their role to include wider practice venues in the "community of care," understanding the language of outcomes will be essential.

To date there is no textbook that addresses this new field. The topic areas in this book are presented together for the first time in the context of clinical laboratory medicine, specifically for practicing clinical laboratorians, pathology residents, medical students, and students of clinical laboratory science. Some background knowledge of laboratory medicine (including basic predictive value theory), basic probability theory, statistics, and study design is assumed on the part of the reader.

Michael G. Bissell, MD, PhD, MPH
Pittsburgh, Pennsylvania

List of Contributors

Raymond D. Aller, MD
Director, MDS Laboratories
Atlanta, Georgia

Larry H. Bernstein, MD
Section Chief, Chemistry,
  Coagulation, Transfusion
  Medicine
Department of Pathology
Bridgeport Hospital
Yale New Haven Health
Bridgeport, Connecticut

Michael G. Bissell, MD, PhD, MPH
Professor of Pathology,
  MCP/Hahnemann University
  School of Medicine and
  Director of Clinical Pathology
Allegheny General Hospital
Pittsburgh, Pennsylvania

D. Joe Boone, PhD
Assistant Director for Science
Division of Laboratory Systems
U.S. Centers for Disease Control
  and Prevention (CDC)
Atlanta, Georgia

Stephen Brossette, PhD
MS IV and Medical Scientist
  Training Program Fellow
University of Alabama
  Birmingham School of Medicine
Birmingham, Alabama

Diane Francis, MPH
Laboratory Assurance Program
Graduate School of Public Health
San Diego State University
San Diego, California

Louise K. Hofherr, PhD
Laboratory Assurance Program
Graduate School of Public Health
San Diego State University
San Diego, California

Catarina I. Kiefe, PhD, MD
Professor, Department of
  Preventive Medicine,
School of Medicine,
University of Alabama at
  Birmingham,
Birmingham, Alabama

Stephen T. Mennemeyer, PhD
Associate Professor
Department of Health Care
  Organization and Policy
School of Public Health
University of Alabama at
  Birmingham
Birmingham, Alabama

Stephen A. Moser, PhD
Associate Professor
Department of Pathology
University of Alabama Birmingham
Birmingham, Alabama

K. Michael Peddecord, DrPH
Professor
Graduate School of Public Health
San Diego State University
San Diego, California

Stephen R. Raab, MD
Professor of Pathology,
    MCP/Hahnemann University
    School of Medicine and
    Director of Cytopathology and
    Outcomes Research
Allegheny General Hospital
Pittsburgh, Pennsylvania

Marc Silverstein, MD
Director, Center for Healthcare
    Research
Medical University of South
    Carolina
Charleston, South Carolina

James W. Winkelman, MD
Vice President for Laboratories,
    Brigham and Women's Hospital,
Boston, Massachusetts
Professor of Pathology
Harvard University Medical School
Boston, Massachusetts

The Patient Outcomes Movement in Relation to Laboratory Medicine: History, Economics, Concepts

Chapter 1

Introduction: What's in a Laboratory Outcome?

M. G. Bissell

HISTORICAL BACKGROUND

The current interest in measuring patient outcomes is best understood in the context of the history and economics of the evolving U.S. health-care system. At the close of the nineteenth century, allopathic medicine, politically dominant over its rival schools, was initially operated under a professional model as a hospital- and clinic-centered fee-for-service enterprise (Starr, 1982). Medicine was first forced to assess its own quality and value by the work of such pioneers as surgeon Ernest Codman. Codman (whose work eventually led to the founding of the Joint Commission on Accreditation of Health Care Organizations, JCAHO) envisioned a system of quality assessment based on how patients *did*, after surgery for instance (Iezzoni,1997). Given the sociology and economics of organized medicine at the time, however, Codman's *outcomes*-based approach was politically unpopular with his colleagues and was replaced by a *structural* model of quality and value, based on the formal qualifications and training of the staff and the nature of the physical facilities. This approach was inspired to some degree by the report of the Flexner Commission on medical education (Starr, 1982).

Eventually, the structural approach came under internal pressure from growth in specialization, the size and complexity of the health-care team, new emphasis on technology, and reimbursement driven by procedures. It thus next broadened into a system that included an important emphasis on measurement of the efficiency of various production *processes* within the hospital. Today, in the economic environment of prepayment, capitation, managed care. and a heightened overall concern for the determination of "value added" in health-care, the outcomes approach has been rediscovered, and is rapidly becoming the dominant model. The structural- and process-based approaches, however, have left behind a major conceptual legacy that thoroughly permeates the practice of modern laboratory medicine (Bissell et al., 1994).

Hospital-based laboratorians are generally well versed in basic statistics and are indeed quite familiar with certain process-based statistical quality control methods (like process control charts and ROC curves) that are still somewhat novel (but rapidly becoming standard) to other professional groups in the new environment. Furthermore, the ideas of quality assessment via proficiency surveys and of external benchmarking ("report cards") are not at all new to laboratory medicine as they are to many other hospital services. These portions of the legacy of process-based thinking will be useful to hospital laboratorians as they negotiate the transition to the new world of outcomes. The major skill set lacking from their conceptual armamentarium (though often not from that of their laboratorian colleagues in public health) is an understanding of the basic fundamentals of the population-based study of human disease. The "basic science" of the outcomes-based approach is clinical epidemiology, an area encompassing statistical characterization of human populations, epidemiological measures of disease occurrence, and the fundamentals of population-based study design.

The first major health-care sector to become proficient in an outcomes-based approach to its own economics was the pharmaceutical industry. Faced with separate federal regulation under the U.S. Food and Drug Act, pharmaceutical firms early on became heavily involved in the evolution and development of the field of clinical trials design for the determination of the safety and efficacy of drugs. Thus, even before widespread interest in health-care reform began to surface, pharmaceutical firms were extremely well positioned to broaden their clinical trials-based outcomes expertise to include assessment of the economic value of their products. This field, called pharmacoeconomics, thus provides examples of outcomes studies that are conceptually and methodologically instructive for laboratorians (Spilker,1991).

While drug treatment outcomes have been rigorously evaluated for some time, diagnostic tests and procedures have not. Clinical best practices in laboratory use remain less certain. Laboratory-related outcomes analysis can reduce this uncertainty, define appropriate utilization and value, and perhaps even help evolve new roles for the clinical laboratory in the health-care enterprise. In the current health-care economic environment, with its new emphasis on outcomes, there is now great sensitivity to the costs associated with "little ticket" ancillary items like laboratory tests. This new questioning of laboratory utilization rates has led to recent estimates that much of all clinical laboratory testing may be "unnecessary." So far, of course, these statements are being made in the absence of any significant body of work relating laboratory utilization to patient outcomes. At the outset of the creation of this necessary body of work, it is important to avoid the "diagnostic nihilism" potentially implicit in today's estimates of presumed laboratory overutilization. One way to do so is to revisit laboratory medicine's historical "track record" with regard to its impact on the incidence and prevalence of disease. A major example is the routine use of the screening Pap smear, which since its widespread introduction has been associated with a worldwide decrease in cervical cancer mortality (see Raab, Chapter 11).

ECONOMIC BACKGROUND

To understand the economics of the clinical laboratory industry, one must start with the question: Who buys health care? The answer is that for all compensated care, and in roughly equal proportions, the final check is written by a federal agency, by an insurance carrier, or by the patient's household. The dollars used by federal agencies are tax dollars, the dollars used by insurance carriers are, for the most part, shifted from cash wages to benefits, and, of course, direct pay is directly out of pocket. Thus, it is the ultimate consumers, patients and their households, who actually buy health care (Reinhardt, 1993). This is important because all attempts to place a value on component health-care services must do so from the perspective of the purchaser. If employers, for example, are regarded as the purchaser, this valuation may very well differ importantly from that of the recipients of care.

What do health-care consumers buy? They do not directly buy component goods and services (bed days, doctor visits, inpatient drugs, laboratory tests). They do buy medical interventions or encounters with the health-care system for purposes of diagnosing, treating, or preventing illness episodes. The cost to U.S. consumers of the health care they buy currently exceeds a trillion dollars per annum (Levit et al., 1998).

What drives the increases in this cost? It appears to have been mostly a matter of greater intensity of service rather than greater frequency of service; i.e., there has been a long-term increase in the expenditures per patient day and per visit rather than in the number or length of visits. The cost driver appears to have been common to both fee-for-service and health maintenance organization (HMO) environments and to have existed in a variety of different developed countries with widely differing health-care systems in place. Many economists believe that the most likely cost driver is inelastic consumer demand for more and newer medical technology.

This presents an interesting contrast with the rest of the economy. In U.S. health care historically, the test of any medical innovation has been solely whether or not it produces favorable outcomes, not whether those outcomes have been worth the cost. In the rest of the economy, cost has always been a factor in whether or not an innovation succeeds. Thus in vitro diagnostic tests, for example, have been introduced and used historically without the economic cost test ever being applied. National patterns of laboratory test utilization reflect this history: In vitro diagnostic testing represented about $30 billion, or approximately 5% of total health care expenditures in 1993, double the amount in 1985 (Bissell et al., 1994). Now that the cost test is being applied, the question has become: What patient outcomes are we getting for the cost of laboratory tests?

Up to now, the value of laboratory services has often been defined de facto in terms of a laboratory's "quality," but in the new economic environment we must ask: What is laboratory quality and from whose perspective is it defined? How much does it cost? What is it worth? Who will determine it, and how will they do this? Quality in health care generally is defined by the Joint Commission on Accreditation of Health Care Organizations (JCAHO) as "the degree to which patient care services increase the probability of desired patient outcomes and reduce the probability of undesired outcomes, given the current state of knowledge" (JCAHO, 1996). The performance of a laboratory should, then, be measured in terms of patient outcomes and cost, which then give rise to judgments of benefit (or utility) and value, where:

Value = k × [Utility/Cost]

One further dimension in the determination of value involves the basic distinction between laboratory data and laboratory information. If we enumerate the elements of value in laboratory data we find that that they form a familiar litany: the right result, on the right patient, at the right time, in the right form, for the right price, per customer specifications. Elements of value in laboratory information, on the other hand, sound right, but are less commonly and uniformly present: the right test choice, referred to the right reference range, with the right interpretation, with the right awareness of the test's limitations, with the right advice as to what to do next with the result, with the right knowledge of when testing is completed, with the right understanding of the clinical context of testing.

For a test to be of diagnostic value to a patient, for example, it must convey information in the sense that it can change the physician's estimate of the probability of disease. It must be able to change this probability estimate enough to affect subsequent patient management decisions and have a sufficiently high expected value to outweigh any risk involved in the performance of the test itself. The *expected value of clinical information*, by the way, is a technical term in decision theory that represents the difference between the health outcome with the test and without the test, estimated using a decision tree for the clinical workup involved. It is a concept that is explored more fully in texts on decision analysis (e.g., Weinstein and Fineberg, 1980).

THE CONCEPTUAL BASICS OF LABORATORY-RELATED OUTCOMES

Outcomes can be defined as the results of medical interventions, in terms of either health or cost. *Patient outcomes* are the results of medical care on a patient's well-being, in terms that are perceptible to the patient, including such things as functional status, health status, and quality of life. Examples of commonly used *outcomes measures* include: mortality, morbidity, quality-of-life measures, satisfaction with care, cost of care, length of stay, work days lost, complication rate, nosocomial infection rate, and readmission rate. Health status measures are typically tracked as defect rates, measures of patient satisfaction as the answer to the survey question "would you return here for future care or recommend this institution to another?," and cost as dollars of expense. Outcomes measures are typically analyzed by determining the expected number of occurrences (E) for each risk class studied, and subtracting this from the number of observed occurrences (A). This difference (A – E) is then summed across all risk classes (Beck, 1997).

Laboratory-related outcomes should be thought of as including not only direct effects of testing, but also indirect effects on the timing, efficiency, and satisfaction of overall patient care. David Eddy defines three levels of laboratory-related patient outcomes. The *first-order laboratory outcome* is simply the probability of a given test result, i.e., the performance (sensitivity, specificity) of the test in actual practice. Thus every test has at least four sets of outcomes associated with it, namely, the consequences of a true positive, a true negative, a false positive, and a false negative result. The *second-order laboratory outcome* is the probability of disease or abnormality in the patient vis-à-vis the test result as estimated by the caregiver receiving the laboratory result, e.g., the predictive value of the test as determined using Bayes' theorem. The *third-order laboratory outcome* is the actual probability of a change in health status of the patient resulting from any therapeutic interventions either instituted or foregone based on the test result (Eddy, 1997).

Thus the real effect of a test is measured as the change in probabilities of health outcomes and depends on the patient population being tested. It also depends on what would be done if the test were not available, and cannot be determined without knowing the outcomes of any treatment decisions that follow it. Studies of true laboratory-related outcomes would ideally include clinical trials as a definitive methodology. But such trials must be conducted in such a way that all positive and negative test results would be invariably acted upon as such. Since this is seldom possible in actual practice, these studies must often of necessity be built up from models and indirect evidence.

In practice, there are often major problems when studying outcomes. These measurements are not value-neutral, people's jobs sometimes are on the line, and people's quality of life is always on the line. Outcomes studies require, but often lack, a unified focus, what with the typical necessity of using data originally collected for other purposes. There is typically a considerable cost (in dollars and person hours) associated with capturing outcomes data. This has been due, in part, to the lack of a standardized data dictionary available to workers in this field. There also is a basic question about how to analyze outcomes data: to risk adjust or not to risk adjust (The concept of risk adjustment will be further defined in the chapter on clinical epidemiology.) Finally, there are the political issues connected with identifying individual providers in outcomes studies (Beck, 1997).

The quality of a potential outcomes measure has several critical dimensions. The first of these is its *relevance* to real-world questions, the likelihood of continuing applicability or pertinence of the measure over time. The *reliability* of an outcomes measure is its reproducibility, i.e., the accuracy and consistency of the application of data elements, as well as its ability to identify the events it was designed to measure, across multiple study settings. The *validity* of a measure is the extent to which it raises good questions about the quality of care and indicates opportunities for improvement. A measure's *discrimination* is the extent to which it demonstrates significant variation in performance in multiple study settings. A variety of standardized outcomes measurement instruments have been developed that have potential application in the study of laboratory-related outcomes, including the JCAHO IMSystem, the NCQA HEDIS 3.0, the University of Wisconsin Minimum Data Set (MDS), the Medical Outcomes Trust Short Form (SF) 36, the University of Colorado Outcomes and Assessment Information Set (OASIS), the Acute Physiology and Chronic Health Evaluation (APACHE) critical care severity measures, the Picker Institute Patient Satisfaction Index, the Florida Institute of Medicine rehabilitation Measures, and the Maryland Hospital Project (Beck, 1997).

The statistical analysis of an outcomes study should include the following. The choice of any adjustment techniques used in the analysis should be clearly justified and understandable. Sample size must be adequate to provide the statistical power necessary for valid conclusions. Any statistical techniques used to aggregate data across studies must be used appropriately. Confidence intervals should be well defined and clearly stated on all summary statistics. Finally, sensitivity analysis or other measures of the validity of the results for the intended use should be provided.

Understanding laboratory-related outcomes, moreover, enables the clinical laboratory to become involved with institutional process improvement, including practice guidelines development, redesign of laboratory services, and application of patient satisfaction measures within the institution. It also may hold the potential for the laboratory to become more directly involved with patients themselves. A major potential application for outcomes assessment is its use as a basis for real-time clinical decision support both for providers and for patients. For providers, having real-time access to epidemiologic databases of laboratory results related to patient outcomes, perhaps searchable by expert systems, can provide customized solutions to problems of empiric treatment. For patients, focused, thorough, and unbiased education based on outcomes can facilitate truly informed decision making in those (increasingly numerous) situations in which the patient's preferences are critical.

A *clinical process* is a series of linked steps, often sequential, intended to cause a set of outcomes to occur, transform resource inputs into outputs, generate useful information, and add value. Managing a clinical process starts with knowledge of processes, their interactions (systems), human psychology, sources of variation, and a system for ongoing learning. Process management is directly analogous to scientific method. Continuous improvement (e.g., total quality management [TQM], PDCA cycle, etc.), like research, is based on hypothesis and test. Quality and cost are linked. Changing one affects the other; similarly, cost affects access. The outcomes movement is one aspect of the contemporary effort to demonstrate and improve the value of patient care by introducing greater standardization and accountability in the management of clinical processes.

Clinical practice guidelines, pathways, and parameters are the institutional expression of this effort. They can be thought of as *case management systems* to control cost outcomes or as *research systems* for continuous learning to improve medical outcomes. When these more standardized approaches to care are implemented, their use and effectiveness are typically monitored carefully and validated through the follow-up of patient outcomes. Ideally, guidelines are initially developed based on the results of studies of the outcomes of each component patient intervention. Thus, they are part of a dynamic process in which ongoing assessment and management of outcomes is a fundamental part. Understanding laboratory-related patient outcomes enables the active participation of the clinical laboratory in this process.

REFERENCES

Beck JR. Pathologist as designer of process improvement. *CAP Foundation Conference VIII. Patient-centered pathology practice: Outcomes and Accountability.* St. Petersburg, FL, Jan. 30–Feb. 2, 1997.

Bissell MG and the National Affairs Committee of CLMA. Ensuring universal access to quality laboratory services: CLMA white paper. *Clin. Lab. Manage. Rev.* 1994;8:185–240.

Eddy DM. What every pathologist should know about outcomes. *CAP Foundation ConferenceVIII. Patient-centered pathology practice: Outcomes and Accountability.* St. Petersburg, FL, Jan. 30–Feb. 2, 1997.

Iezzoni LI (ed.). *Risk Adjustment for Measuring Healthcare Outcomes,* second edition. Health Administration Press, Chicago, 1997.

Joint Commission on Accreditation of Health Care Organizations. *Comprehensive Accreditation Manual for Pathology and Laboratory Services.* JCAHO, Oakbrook Terrace, IL, 1996.

Levit KR, Lazenby HC, Braden BR, and National Health Accounts Team. National Health Spending Trends in 1996. *Health Affairs* 1998;17(1).

Reinhardt UE. Reorganizing the financial flows in American health care. *Health Affairs* 1993;12 Suppl:172–193.

Spilker B. Pharmacoeconomic trials. Chapter 42 in *Guide to Clinical Trials*. Raven Press, New York, 1991.

Starr P. *The Social Transformation of American Medicine*. Basic Books, New York, 1982.

Weinstein MC, Fineberg HV. *Clinical Decision Analysis*. W. B. Saunders, Philadelphia, 1980.

Chapter 2

Laboratory Services: A Health Services Research Perspective

M. D. Silverstein

Health services research is an interdisciplinary field that addresses access, organization, financing, quality, cost, and outcomes of care. A health services research perspective on laboratory services requires an assessment of cost of laboratory services, quality of laboratory services, and access to laboratory services. Most laboratorians would appropriately agree that there are few barriers to access to laboratory services, which are provided in high volume with high degrees of accuracy at high efficiency and relatively low cost. Yet there is increased scrutiny of laboratory services and a need for laboratorians to evaluate the role of laboratory services in patient outcomes. Laboratorians, therefore, need to be familiar with measures and the value of laboratory services in providing information that lead to diagnoses, changes in treatment, and improvements in patient outcomes.

A future need for health services research studies of laboratory services must focus on the development of measures of the value of information obtained from laboratory tests. Information from laboratory tests is potentially valuable to individual patients in improving understanding of the nature and the prognosis of clinical course of an illness, to managers in the health care system, to investigators in providing information on the scientific understanding of disease, and finally to public health workers for population surveillance of disease.

Health services research is a newly recognized interdisciplinary field of inquiry. Health services research has been defined by the Institute of Medicine as a "multidisciplinary field of inquiry, both basic and applied, that examines the use, costs, quality, accessibility, delivery, organization, financing, and outcomes of health care services to increase knowledge and understanding of the structure, processes, and effects of health services for individuals and populations" (Field et al., 1995).

While health services research is not a new field, it has obtained increasing importance in recent years because of rising health-care costs, wide variations in the use of services, and concerns about the quality of care and the increasing numbers of uninsured and underinsured Americans who have limited access to care. All these issues have potential impact on patient outcomes. Laboratorians' professional interests require an understanding of health services research and its implications for laboratory services.

Three major health services research themes in the 1990s that are likely to continue as major issues into the next millennium are cost of care, quality of care, and access to care. Healthcare costs have risen markedly in recent years. Currently, U.S. health-care costs are over $1 trillion and represent over 14% of the U.S. gross domestic product (GDP). There has been some reduction in the rapid double-digit annual increase in health-care costs. In 1996, the most recent year for which data are available, the increase in health-care cost was only 4.4% (Levit et al., 1998). The increase in health-care costs cannot be sustained and has severely constrained the ability of the federal government, state governments, and private employers to pay for health-care costs. In response to the increase in health-care costs there has been vertical and horizontal consolidation in the health-care industry as well as striking growth in managed care. These changes have had substantial impacts on clinical laboratories. While laboratories have adopted new technologies and new management practices to control cost, it is very likely that cost concerns will increase in the future.

A second theme in health services research is quality of care. There have been a variety of studies that have documented widespread variations in the use of medical procedures and laboratory tests. These variations have been quite large, far beyond that expected to be explained by variations in the incidence or prevalence of disease in a population. One manifestation of these variations has been the large number of studies that attempt to modify physicians' test ordering to reduce the use of laboratory services. These studies have been predicated upon the notion that some part of the current pattern in use of laboratory services is discretionary and can be reduced without adverse effect on patient care (Kaplan et al., 1985; Narr et al., 1991; Narr et al., 1997; Turnbull and Buck, 1987).

For laboratorians, the most striking initiative relevant to issues in quality of care is the Clinical Laboratory Improvement Amendments of 1988 (CLIA'88). CLIA had an impact on both the costs and quality of laboratory tests. In its effort to ensure high quality of diagnostic laboratory tests for humans, Congress enacted CLIA'88 seemingly without recognizing the increase in costs to laboratories that have resulted from need to follow the requirements of CLIA. Complex Medicare rules regarding specific justifications ("medical necessity") for tests and the separate ordering of tests that have been bundled may further increase costs to laboratories, and ultimately to payers of health care.

The third health services issue is access to care. Access to care is generally operationalized as lack of health insurance. In 1997, there were over 40 million Americans who were uninsured and larger numbers of Americans are believed to be underinsured. Laboratory services, however, are generally not expensive compared to other health services, and indeed most insurance, including Medicaid, covers laboratory services. While some fee schedules may not provide adequate coverage to pay for the cost of some laboratory tests, in general, costs of individual laboratory tests are not a major component of health-care costs. Thus it would appear that costs of laboratory services should not be a major concern for health services research. Although the individual costs of laboratory tests are small, the large volume of testing does result in high aggregate costs. Laboratorians would rightly indicate that laboratory tests cost only a small fraction of all health-care costs. Nevertheless, in an era with widespread concerns about health-care costs, it is not reasonable to expect laboratories to escape pressures to reduce health-care costs.

Laboratorians can benefit by understanding a health services research perspective on laboratory services. Laboratorians can also benefit by using a conceptual framework for measuring the value of laboratory services. Clinical laboratories are in many ways similar to diagnostic radiology: Both areas provide information on structure and function that can be used by clinical laboratorians and radiologists as well as other clinicians in establishing diagnoses. The diagnostic information provided by laboratory services and imaging services can be measured by its ability to make new diagnoses, change treatment, and thereby improve patient outcomes.

This was the basis of a conceptual framework first suggested by Fryback and Thornberry for application to diagnostic imaging (Fryback and Thornbury, 1991) and adapted by Silverstein and Boland (1994) for the evaluation of laboratory tests. In this framework the key issues are the ability of the laboratory services to make accurate and reproducible measures of the analytes that lead to sensitive and specific tests to establish a diagnosis. New diagnoses are the basis of physicians' decisions to initiate therapeutic or preventive interventions that will beneficially affect the clinical course of disease and patient outcomes (Boland et al., 1996).

In addition to the conceptual framework for evaluating the effectiveness of laboratory services in contributing to patient outcomes, laboratorians and health services researchers may benefit from additional measures of the value of information to patients, to the health-care system, and to the population. Information about health obtained from laboratory tests may be highly valued by patients, physicians, and other providers even if it doesn't lead to a change in diagnosis, change in treatment, or change in outcome. Some patients value information because of the understanding it can provide of the etiology of disease, the reassurance that may come if disease is not present, or the information about the future course of an illness that may result from the prognostic information of laboratory testing. The health-care system may find information about the overall burden of disease in a population based screening program. Finally, the population may benefit from increased understanding through public health programs that can result from surveillance of patterns of disease or the genetic predisposition to disease in a population. Laboratorians generally have not had good measures or adequate studies of the value of the information to individual persons, to health-care systems, or to populations. A future agenda for health services research or laboratory services must deal with development of measures of the value of information, in addition to better study of the role of laboratory services in establishing diagnoses, in changing treatments, and in changing patient outcomes.

REFERENCES

Boland BJ, Wollan PC, Silverstein MD. Yield of laboratory tests for case-finding in the ambulatory general medical examination. *Am J Med* 1996;101:142–152

Field MJ, Tranquada RE, Feasley JC, et al. *Health Services Research: Work Force and Educational issues*. National Academy Press, Washington, DC, 1995.

Fryback DG, Thornbury JR. The efficacy of diagnostic imaging. *Med Decision Making* 1991;11:88–94.

Kaplan EB, Sheiner LB, Boeckmann AJ, Roisen MF, Beal SL, Cohen SN, Nicoll CD. The usefulness of preoperative laboratory screening. *J Am Med Assoc* 1985;253:3576–3581.

Levit KR, Lazenby HC, Braden BR, and National Health Accounts Team. National health spending trends in 1996. *Health Affairs* 1998;17(1).

Narr BJ, Hensen TR, Warner MA. Preoperative laboratory screening in healthy Mayo patients: Cost effective elimination of tests and unchanged outcomes. *Mayo Clin. Proc.* 1991;66:155–159.

Narr BJ, Warner ME, Schroeder DR, Warner MA. Outcomes of patients with no laboratory assessment before anesthesia and a surgical procedure. *Mayo Clin. Proc.* 1997;72:505–509.

Silverstein MD, Boland BJ. Conceptual framework for evaluating laboratory tests: Case-finding in ambulatory patients. *Clin. Chem.* 1994;40(8):1621–1627.

Turnbull JM, Buck C. The value of preoperative screening investigations in otherwise healthy individuals. *Arch. Intern. Med.* 1987;147:1101–1105.

Chapter 3

Initiatives in Laboratory-Related Outcomes Research

D. J. Boone

Americans have always been a pragmatic people. As much as we like the bells and whistles of our car, cell phone, or computer, we are ultimately interested in a very fundamental question. We want to know if the device we have chosen does what it is supposed to do or not. With this general outlook on life, it is little wonder that Americans are questioning the value of the health-care services they receive. While they can readily evaluate for themselves their ability to access health-care services and have an increasing awareness of how much these services cost, they are often not able to determine whether the quality of care they would receive from provider X would be better than that from provider Y. A sense of frustration with usual medical practice seems to be emerging among citizens, which has led more than 40% of the public to attempt to go beyond traditional medical practice and actively seek out their own cures for what they think ails them (Jonas, 1998). What is somewhat surprising about the huge investment Americans are making in personal alternatives to traditional medicine is that there is little scientific evidence that these alternatives work. In addition, there is tremendous variability in some of the natural products being used, and practitioners of alternative medicine are not certified or licensed by anyone. Does this willingness to accept less scientific proof for these alternatives portend a change in public attitudes?

In addition to the growing trend of the public to seek their own treatment alternatives, another area of rapid growth has been in their ability to perform or obtain their own laboratory tests. In some cases this trend has encompassed the worried-well wanting to determine their risk of heart disease, but more recently patients are self-monitoring their diabetes and anticoagulant therapy. Many of these products are useful tools to assist

15

practitioners in delivery of cost-effective patient care and are tributes to the skill of the diagnostics industry. In this chapter we review some of the initiatives undertaken by various government agencies, professional organizations, and industry to demonstrate that certain laboratory tests or practices do indeed make a difference in patient outcome. We explore factors that make evidence-based research in this area difficult and we examine what might be done in the future to ensure that the contributions laboratory medicine can make to patient care are more fully realized.

At the outset, it should be stated that the need for better definitions and measures for outcomes related to laboratory medicine has hampered research in this area. Clinical outcome has rarely been measured. This has lead to an emphasis on studies that evaluate the impact of changes in the structure or processes involved in delivery of laboratory service on access to or cost of service, rather than direct measures of patient outcome (Witte, 1994). Soon after the passage of the Clinical Laboratory Improvement Amendments of 1998 (CLIA'88) (PL 100–578 USC 201, 1988), the Centers for Disease Control and Prevention (CDC) was delegated responsibility for conducting studies to examine the relationship between laboratory practice and the accuracy and reliability of test results. This encompasses the structure and processes employed in the provision of laboratory service. In terms of laboratory practice, the time required to access services, the quality of the information generated, the total cost of service delivery, and patient outcomes are all clearly relevant measures. If performance of a laboratory test and placing the results in the hands of an educated health-care provider is viewed as a medical intervention, then the relationship between laboratory service and outcomes is easier to define. Unfortunately, the laboratory may be very remote from both the health-care provider and the patient, may not have been consulted or informed in any way about the purpose for testing, and often does not know about a patient's outcome. It is the indirect involvement with provision of patient care and all the potentially confounding variables associated with actual patient care delivery that make the direct link between patient outcome and provision of laboratory services difficult to evaluate.

Despite these difficulties, the Centers for Disease Control and Prevention (CDC) began working with the College of American Pathologists (CAP) in 1989 to develop a series of projects to measure impact of critical laboratory practices on patient outcome. For example, in 1991, a blood bank survey was sent to participants in the CAP Transfusion Medicine Surveys Program to explore the relationship between active surveillance to detect and correct defects in 24 risk-prone steps in the transfusion process and the number and type of complications associated with the transfusion service (Boone et al., 1995). Although monitoring of specific risk-prone steps in the transfusion process could not be directly linked with prevention of the complications studied, active surveillance is more likely to focus attention on defect-prone processes and provide greater opportunity for improved patient outcome. An additional project conducted by the CAP/CDC working group examined the impact of intraoperative pathology consultations on patient outcomes (Zarbo et al., 1996). In this, pathologists from 472 participating institutions selected 20 consecutive intraoperative consultations and established the five most common indications for obtaining the surgical consult and whether the information provided modified, terminated, or initiated surgical procedures. Regardless of the initial indication, these consultations were found to change surgical procedures in an average of 39% of the 9164 cases examined. The preliminary results of another study conducted by the CAP/CDC working group led Schifman, Pindar, and Bryan (1997) to conduct a randomized case control study comparing standard microbiology reporting with targeted reporting for antimicrobial susceptibility testing. The target approach involving a laboratory-based process to integrate pharmacy, laboratory, and clinician data, leading to rapid notification of the clinician when the antimicrobial susceptibility test results and antibiotic therapy were discordant. Reviewing 254 cases, discordance between test results and antibiotic therapy was detected in 55% of patients and confirmed after clinical review in 19%. Patients were placed on appropriate antibiotic therapy significantly sooner and at higher rates with targeted notification than with standard reporting procedures.

Given the difficulty of demonstrating a direct link between patient outcome and parameters of the quality of laboratory service provided, innovative research approaches are required. Mennemeyer and Winkelman (1993) described a method they termed downstream event monitoring in which they reviewed mountains of Medicare claims data looking for a significant increase in adverse patient outcome, such as stroke and myocardial infarction, soon after a laboratory test for prothrombin time. Adverse patient outcome seemed to be associated with performance of less than 40 tests/month, switching from one laboratory to another, not having had a test within the last 6 months, and the laboratory being located in a state with less rigorous laboratory regulations. The etiology of these associations remains to be determined. If the associations can be demonstrated to be real, this technique will provide an additional means to identify laboratories whose poor performance may jeopardize patient care. The authors are attempting to replicate, using data on tests performed by hospital laboratories on an outpatient basis, the results of their earlier study, which was based on data only from independent and physician office laboratories (Mennemeyer,1998). The authors report on this work elsewhere in this volume.

In 1994, the CDC funded the Ambulatory Sentinel Practice Network (ASPN) to examine the nature of problems associated with laboratory services in the delivery of primary care (Nutting et al., 1996). A crude rate of 1.1 problems with laboratory testing per 100 patient visits was found. The most commonly encountered problems involved test ordering and specimen handling (56%), while 13% of the problems were associated with the analysis itself. Of the problems that were found, the physician judged 27% as affecting either the diagnosis or treatment of the patient

Historically, funding for laboratory-based outcome research has been difficult to obtain. In 1994, the American Association for Clinical Chemistry (AACC) secured funding to initiate some small-scale outcome research studies. In 1995, the CDC initiated an Investigational Consortium for Research in Laboratory Medicine, which was aimed at increasing the capability of laboratorians and clinicians to engage in outcome-based laboratory medicine research. The Mayo Clinic, the Clinical Laboratory Management Association (CLMA), and the University of Alabama at Birmingham were each awarded a cooperative agreement. The hope was that an ongoing laboratory medicine research program would evolve from these initial efforts. The CLMA supported four independent investigations (Bissell et al., 1998). One was a study at the Medical College of Virginia that evaluated the clinical and financial benefits of adding an automated cardiac Troponin I assay to their existing cardiac panel. Although not designed as a randomized clinical trial, Anderson et al. (1998) were able to demonstrate that adding cardiac Troponin I decreased length of stay for patients classified as low risk for acute myocardial infarction, thereby lowering total and variable hospital costs. In a second investigation, Barr and Otto (1998) selected a National Committee for Clinical Laboratory Standards (NCCLS) document, "Ancillary (Bedside) Blood Glucose Testing in Acute and Chronic Care Facilities, C-30." Using a Delphi process, the authors developed a scoring instrument to evaluate bedside glucose monitoring in 14 general hospitals in the Boston area. They were able to rank these institutions using the instrument, but did not attempt to examine the relationship between scores on their instrument and patient outcomes. In a prospective randomized trial, Steinberger and Hanson (1998) examined the rate of arrhythmias in postoperative cardiac surgical patients when magnesium replacement was monitored using either measurement of ionized magnesium or total magnesium. They found no difference in postoperative management of cardiopulmonary bypass patients when either of these measures of magnesium replacement was used. Based on their unexpected findings, Steinberger and Hanson advocate an outcomes-based justification before introducing new laboratory tests. Finally, Zinn (1998) used a Delphi technique to develop a consensus for performance areas and indicators of performance. These tools might eventually be useful in self-assessment of such laboratory service factors as information systems, test ordering/utilization, efficiency of diagnosis and treatment, outcome assessment, and customer satisfaction.

At the January 8, 1997, Clinical Laboratory Improvement Advisory Committee meeting, Dr. George Klee reported on work on one of three projects being carried out at Mayo Clinic Laboratories, which demonstrates the critical need for defining analytical precision and accuracy goals (Klee, 1997). Laboratory research has often focused on the analytical precision goals for testing, and Dr. Klee has investigated the utility of defining analytical accuracy or bias goals. Small shifts in the accuracy of calcium, thyroid-stimulating hormone, and prostate specific antigen tests can have potentially adverse effects on the diagnosis and treatment of large groups of patients. Improved detection and prevention of these small but significant shifts will require better quality control (QC) and quality assurance (QA) approaches and may also be dependent upon having more accurate and robust test systems. An additional study was aimed at prospectively determining the diagnostic and clinical yield for evaluation and management of arterial hypertension when a patient is found to have an abnormal test result such as an elevated creatinine, low potassium, elevated urinary metanephrines, or elevated aldosterone. Finally, the value of providing diabetic patients with a laboratory summary sheet designed specifically to assist them with managing their own glucose control was evaluated and this was found to be a useful tool to improve control of diabetes.

The value of point-of-care (POC) testing in expediting a change in treatment was evaluated by investigators at the University of Alabama at Birmingham (UAB) (Kilgore et al., 1998). They compared centralized versus distributed methods for delivering "stat" test results for blood gas, glucose, and electrolyte assays. The parameters for comparison included: (a) laboratory turnaround time (TAT), (b) therapeutic TAT, and (c) staff satisfaction. Therapeutic TAT, defined as the time from the initiating order to the receipt of the result and the implementation of any indicated change in treatment, was obtained by direct observation of testing procedures at the bedside and timing each step in the process. Observing therapeutic TAT provided information on the impact of the method of service delivery on clinical decision making. Therapeutic TAT was 12 min shorter for bedside testing compared with a satellite laboratory and 14 min shorter in the satellite laboratory compared with centralized testing. Satellite laboratories received the highest staff satisfaction scores, followed by bedside testing, with the central laboratory receiving the lowest scores. Another UAB study used patient satisfaction as an indicator of quality in evaluating POC laboratory service compared to central laboratory service (Kilgore et al., 1997). The authors describe their rationale for using this approach and specific techniques for developing questionnaires, collecting survey response data, and building a database for analysis. They also address problems that arise in incorporating data from medical records into a research database and the linkage of records from disparate sources. Approaches to cost analysis are discussed, including problems with the use of financial and billing records. Their preliminary results show no significant effects of using POC prothrombin time testing on the overall care of hospital inpatients. Using laboratory charges and total reimbursements for treatment as proxies for cost, they found a significant difference ($p < .0001$) in the cost of POC testing over the cost for testing in the central laboratory.

In a study that could affect the 20,000 patients 50 years of age or older who are scheduled for cataract surgery each year, a Patient Outcomes

Research Team (PORT-II) project funded by the Agency for Health Care Policy and Research (AHCPR) was awarded in 1994 to Johns Hopkins University School of Medicine. They will undertake a 4-year study to determine the value of medical testing prior to cataract surgery. Laboratory medicine parameters included were blood count and electrolytes. This is a rare instance where a randomized clinical trial is being used to develop recommendations on the appropriate use of these tests preoperatively. The principal investigator, Oliver Schein, has shown that there is wide variation in the preoperative use of medical tests internationally (Norregaard et al., 1997).

More examples are emerging illustrating the value of single institution studies as well as those using data across institutions. Mears was able to show that implementing a program of serum prealbumin screening on admission and twice weekly monitoring for protein calorie malnutrition for all adult hospital admissions reduced the length of stay and resulted in significant cost savings to her institution (Mears, 1996). Raab examined the cost-effectiveness of different strategies for rescreening cervical vaginal smears using data obtained from a MEDLINE review and the Surveillance Epidemiology and End Results (SEER) program (Raab, 1998). The results of this study illustrate the fact that different conclusions about effectiveness can be drawn depending on whether the focus is on an individual patient or a patient population.

One of the biggest problems with laboratory-related outcomes research in addition to securing funding has been the lack of a national model. Often the study objectives are not well defined, the findings may only apply to a single institution, and most importantly the results often do not influence medical practice. Thus despite the significant early efforts of the CDC, CAP, AACC, CLMA, and others to develop a sustained laboratory-related outcomes research program, no national-scale program has emerged. In 1996, with financial assistance from Abbott Laboratories, the CLMA developed a research initiative outlining areas of research important to consumers, employers, public health agencies, government regulatory agencies, and healthcare providers as they struggle to find answers to complex questions raised by the changing dynamics of health care delivery in the United States (Steingerger and Hanson, 1998) Current plans call for using the Clinical Laboratory Management Foundation as a vehicle to develop something akin to the Pharmaceutical Research and Manufacturers Association (PhRMA) to serve as a means to plan, fund, and coordinate studies that would address some of the more urgent issues facing laboratory medicine today and into the future. The foundation is envisioned to be a home for academic, professional, and government researchers in a partnership that will allow a pooling of talents to develop research projects that will truly measure patient outcomes and impact national practices and policies directly as the results of studies are disseminated. Through the foundation, researchers will be able to examine the overuse or underuse of a laboratory test and to document improvements in efficiency or effectiveness of care, which are measures of the added value of performing the test. Although both types of research are important in determining where the greatest opportunities are for improving the cost/benefit ratio, the patient is more concerned with how testing will affect his or her own mortality, morbidity, and quality of life. It is these outcomes we all seek to determine. The CLMA Foundation should go a long way in helping the laboratory evaluate its true contributions to the public's health.

REFERENCES

Anderson FP, Fritz ML, Kontos MC, McPherson RA, Jesse RL. Cost-effectiveness of cardiac Troponin I in a systematic chest pain evaluation protocol: Use of Troponin I lowers the length of stay for low-risk cardiac patients. *Clin. Lab. Manage. Rev.* 1998;12(2):63–69.

Barr JT, Otto CN. Development of a quantitative weighted scoring instrument to evaluate bedside glucose testing programs. *Clin. Lab. Manage. Rev.* 1998;12(2):70–79.

Bissell MG et al. CLMA Research Initiative: Moving into the 21st century with leadership in knowledge. *Clin. Lab. Manage. Rev.* 1998;12(4):232–242.

Boone DJ, Steindel SJ, Herron R, Howanitz PJ, Bachner P, Meier F, Schifman R, Zarbo RJ. Transfusion monitoring practices: A study of the College of American Pathologists/Centers for Disease Control and Prevention Outcomes Working Group. *Arch. Pathol. Lab. Med.* 1995;119:999–1006.

Jonas WB. Alternative medicine—Learning from the past, examining the present, advancing the future. *JAMA* 1998;280:1616–1618.

Kilgore ML, Steindel SJ, Smith JA. Using patient satisfaction as an indicator of the quality of laboratory services: Applying social science methods to evaluate outcomes in laboratory medicine. *Clin. Lab. Manage. Rev.* 1997;11(2):93–102.

Kilgore ML, Steindel SJ, Smith JA. Evaluating testing options in an academic health center: Therapeutic turnaround time and staff satisfaction. *Clin. Chem.* 1998;42:1597–1603.

Klee G. http://www.phppo.cdc.gov/dls/claic/claic197.htm Addendum M.

Mears E. Outcomes of continuous process improvement of a nutritional care program incorporating serum prealbumin measurements. *Nutrition* 1996;12(7–8):479–484.

Mennemeyer ST, Winkelman JW. Searching for inaccuracy in clinical laboratory testing using Medicare data: Evidence for prothrombin time. *JAMA* 1993;269:1030–1033.

Mennemeyer ST. Should laboratories be judged by patient outcomes. *Clin. Lab. Manage. Rev.* 1998;12(2):57–62.

Norregaard JC, Schein OD, Anderson GF, Alonso J, Dunn E, Black C, Andersen TF, Bernth-Petersen P, Bellan L, Espallargues M. International variation in ophthalmologic management of patients with cataracts. *Arch. Opthalmol.* 1997;115(3):399–403.

Nutting PA, Main DS, Fischer PM, Stull TM, Pontious M, Seifert M, Boone DJ, Holcomb S. Problems in laboratory testing in primary care. *JAMA* 1996;275:635–639.

Public Law 100–578. Clinical Laboratory Improvement Amendments of 1988. Stat 42 *USC* 201 H.R. 5471, Oct. 31, 1988.

Raab SS. The utility and cost effectiveness of Pap test rescreening. *Clin. Lab. Manage. Rev.* 1998 12(2):91–96.

Schifman RB, Pindar A, Bryan JA. Laboratory practices for reporting bacterial susceptibility tests that affect antibiotic therapy. *Arch. Pathol. Lab. Med.* 1997;121:1168–1170.

Steingerger HA, Hanson CW. Outcome-based justification for implementing new point-of-care tests: There is no difference between magnesium replacement based on ionized magnesium and total magnesium as a predictor of development of arrhythmias in the postoperative cardiac surgical patient. *Clin. Lab. Manage. Rev.* 1998;12(2):87–90.

Witte DL. Defining and measuring outcomes in laboratory medicine: Focus of 1994 Clinical Chemistry Forum. *Clin. Chem. News* 1994;June 2.

Zarbo RJ, Waldemar AS, Bachner P, Howanitz PJ, Meier FA, Schifman RB, Boone DJ, Herron RM, Jr. Indications and immediate patient outcomes of pathology intraoperative consultations: College of American Pathologists/Centers for Disease Control and Prevention Outcomes Working Group. *Arch Pathol Lab Med* 1996;120:19–25.

Zinn J. Use of the Delphi panel method to develop consensus on laboratory performance indicators. *Clin. Lab. Manage. Rev.* 1998;12(2):97–105.

Methodologies for Laboratory-Related Outcomes Study

Chapter 4

Basics of Clinical Epidemiology: Concepts and Terminology

M. G. Bissell

DETERMINING AND ANALYZING DISEASE OCCURRENCE (DIAGNOSIS)

In order to understand the health of a population, it is first necessary to have a clear scheme of diagnostic classification. To describe the occurrence of a disease, it is necessary to determine which individuals have it. This is accomplished by classifying each individual as "diseased" or "disease-free" based on comparing the observations made during a diagnostic examination with diagnostic criteria for the disease being studied. Clinical examination findings are of three general types: symptoms, signs, and tests.

Symptoms are subjective manifestations of disease that only the examined person (patient) may observe, e.g., pain, fatigue, nausea, etc. Symptoms are recorded in the course of taking a clinical history. Note that, due to their subjective nature, symptoms may be described differently by different patients and/or by the same patient at different times. In epidemiologic research, accuracy in recording symptoms is influenced by the means used to collect the data. Standardized methods of interview and questionnaire administration have been developed to increase the reproducibility of this type of data (see chapter 5 on survey research).

Signs are objective manifestations of disease that may be observed by an examiner (usually a physician), e.g., rash, swelling, etc. Signs are observed and recorded in the course of a physical examination. Note that the observation of signs is affected by the subjective judgment of the examiner, as is the interpretation of such diagnostic procedures as auscultation, palpation, x-ray studies, and the examination of tissues. The reproducibility of this type of data (inter- and intra observer reliability) can be increased by standardization of the examination routines and criteria for classification, as well as (in some instances) replacing subjective assessments (e.g., auscultation of heart sounds) with more objective observations (e.g., phonocardiogram).

Tests are objective manifestations of disease that can be read from an analytical instrument and thus are less dependent on subjective judgments on the part of the patient or the examiner, e.g., a blood glucose level. Even with highly standardized measurement techniques, the reproducibility (or imprecision) of laboratory results is subject to variations due to the conditions of obtaining specimens (preanalytic variation) or recording results (postanalytic variation). However, these can be explicitly examined by performing repeated analyses in one laboratory (intralaboratory variation) or by analyzing aliquots in different laboratories (interlaboratory variation) Laboratory measurements may also be subject to bias (inaccuracy), which, however, can also be determined objectively by comparison with a "gold standard" measurement.

Diagnostic criteria are sets of generally agreed upon observations (symptoms, signs, and/or test results) that must be present for a specific diagnosis to be made. The diagnostic criteria thus determine whether or not a given individual is classified as having the disease. Note that formal diagnostic criteria for many diseases are neither well defined nor generally accepted. Also note that disease misclassification can result from diagnostic criteria that are too stringent. In such cases, there will be a small probability that "disease-free" individuals will be classified as "diseased" (false positive rate), but a large probability that "diseased" individuals will be classified as "disease-free" (false negative rate). Similarly, if the diagnostic criteria are not stringent enough, the probability of false positives will be high relative to that of false negatives. Classification of disease is an attempt to systematize the list of known and named diseases. The most widely used such classification is the *International Classification of Disease (ICD),* maintained and regularly updated by the World Health Organization (WHO). The ICD includes 17 main groups of diseases based on their causes, localization, and nature, as follows:

1. Infectious and parasitic diseases
2. Neoplasms
3. Endocrine, nutritional, and metabolic diseases and immune disorders
4. Diseases of the blood and blood-forming organs
5. Mental disorders
6. Diseases of the nervous system and sensory organs
7. Diseases of the circulatory system
8. Diseases of the respiratory system
9. Diseases of the digestive system
10. Diseases of the genitourinary system
11. Complications of pregnancy, childbirth, and the puerperium
12. Diseases of the skin and subcutaneous tissue
13. Diseases of the musculoskeletal system and connective tissue

14. Congenital anomalies
15. Certain conditions originating in the perinatal period
16. Symptoms, signs, and ill-defined conditions
17. Injury and poisoning

Each of these groups contains a great number of specific disease diagnoses that are assigned three-digit code numbers. Note that on each level there are special headings for unclear and unspecified cases. There are also many instances in which two or more diagnoses might apply, which may lead to possible ambiguities when classifying an individual case. There is no completely accurate method to identify all of those individuals who have a certain disease. Diagnostic *accuracy* varies from one disease to another and from one group of individuals to another. Although the objective of epidemiological research is the study of disease occurrence, such studies are actually based on the occurrence of diagnoses. Lack of correspondence between diagnoses and diseases is always a potential source of error in epidemiological research. Knowledge of the different sources of error is essential for the evaluation of epidemiologic studies.

Diagnostic criteria, like individual tests, can be evaluated according to *predictive value theory*. Sensitivity and specificity are two essential quantitative characteristics of diagnostic classifications that allow one to assess the impact of diagnostic error on the measurement of disease occurrence. The *clinical sensitivity* of a disease classification is its "positivity in disease (PID)," i.e., the probability that a "diseased" individual will be correctly classified as "diseased," as follows:

$$\text{Sensitivity} = \frac{\text{number of sick people who are classified as sick}}{\text{total number of sick people}}$$

The *clinical specificity* of a disease classification refers to its "negativity in health (NIH)," i.e., the probability that a "disease-free" individual will be correctly classified as "disease-free," as follows:

$$\text{Sensitivity} = \frac{\text{number of healthy people who are classified as healthy}}{\text{total number of healthy people}}$$

Note that the clinical (or diagnostic) sensitivity and specificity are both proportions. Like probabilities or any other proportions, they are therefore dimensionless quantities that can take on any value between 0 and 1. Also note that these terms should not be confused with *analytical* sensitivity and specificity, which refer to the performance characteristics of chemical analyses and are not proportions.

Predictive values similarly are quantitative characteristics of the diagnostic performance of tests used to screen the population for disease. The *positive predictive value (PV⁺)* of a disease classification scheme is its "rule in capability," i.e., the probability that an individual classified as "diseased" will actually be "diseased," as follows:

$$PV+ = \frac{\text{number of sick people correctly classified}}{\text{total number of sick people}}$$

The *negative predictive value (PV⁻)* of a disease classification scheme is its "rule out capability," i.e., the probability that an individual classified as "disease-free" will actually be "disease-free," as follows:

$$PV- = \frac{\text{number of healthy people correctly classified}}{\text{total number of healthy people}}$$

Critical to population-based medicine is the methodology used in counting disease occurrence. The absolute number of cases of a disease may be useful for some administrative purposes, like determining number and type of facilities needed in a region (Last and Wallace, 1992). More usually in clinical epidemiology, the number of cases of disease is related to a denominator representing the number of individuals in the population from which those cases have arisen. The three most commonly used population measures of disease occurrence are the prevalence, the cumulative incidence, and the incidence rate.

The *prevalence (P)* (also called prevalence rate, prevalence proportion, or point prevalence) is the fraction of the population that is classified as "diseased" at a single point in time. It is numerically equivalent to the probability that an individual subject, randomly chosen from the population, will be correctly classified as "diseased," as follows:

$$P = \frac{\text{number of individuals with disease at time t}}{\text{number of individuals in population at time t}}$$

Note that the prevalence, like a probability or any other proportion, is a dimensionless quantity that may only take on values between 0 and 1. Measures of prevalence may be most relevant in connection with the planning of health services or in assessing the need for medical care in a population. The prevalence of a disease determined by a diagnostic classification with a measured sensitivity and specificity is:

$$P = \frac{P^* + \text{specificity} - 1}{\text{sensitivity} + \text{specificity} - 1}$$

where P* is the total number of individuals classified as "diseased" (= true positives + false positives).

The predictive value (PV$^+$) of a screening test with measured sensitivity and specificity used to classify individuals as "diseased" is a function of these parameters and the prevalence of disease (P), as follows:

$$PV^+ = \frac{P \times \text{ sensitivity}}{P \times \text{ sensitivity} + (1 - P) \times (1 - \text{specificity})}$$

Note: This result is one form of *Bayes' Theorem*. It shows that predictive value will be low when the prevalence is low, even for high values of sensitivity and specificity.

In epidemiologic studies of the cause and/or prevention of disease, the focus is often on the rate at which disease occurs. The term "incidence" describes the frequency of occurrence of new cases during a given time period, i.e., the rate of flow of individuals from the "disease-free" to the "diseased" state, and is expressed in two forms, the cumulative incidence and the incidence rate (Friedman, 1987).

The *cumulative incidence (CI)* (also called cumulative incidence rate and incidence proportion) is the fraction of "nondiseased" subjects who become "diseased" during a specified time period. It represents the average probability of risk of acquiring the disease and is a function of the population size, the "at risk" time period, and the "force of morbidity" driving disease occurrence, i.e., the proportion of individuals in the "disease-free" state at the beginning of the period that move to the "diseased" state during the period. It is thus defined as:

$$CI = \frac{\text{number of individuals who get disease during the time period}}{\text{number of individuals in population at beginning of the time period}}$$

Note that the cumulative incidence is a dimensionless proportion like the prevalence, and that its numerator is a subset of its denominator. Sometimes, in studies covering long time periods, the numerator is corrected by adding back the number of individuals dying of other causes during the period who would otherwise have been expected to get the disease being studied. The CI is a function of the length of the observation period: the longer the period, the greater the CI. Therefore the period at risk must always be reported and interpreted with the CI for it to be meaningful.

The *incidence rate (I)* (also called incidence density) describes the "force of morbidity" driving the occurrence of the disease in the population. The cumulative incidence or overall number of individuals who move from the "disease-free" to the "diseased" state during any period of time is the product of three factors. These are population size, length of the time period during which each individual in the population remains "disease-free" and thus at risk of disease, and this "force of morbidity." The incidence rate is obtained by dividing the number of cases by the product of the time at risk and the size of the population at risk, thus:

$$I = \frac{\text{number of cases of disease that occur in population during a period of time}}{\substack{\text{sum of all individuals in the population over the} \\ \text{length of time at risk of getting the disease}}}$$

Note that the incidence rate, unlike the previous two measures, is not a proportion, since the numerator is the number of cases and the denominator is a period of time expressed in person-time units (e.g., "person-years," "person-months," etc.). Thus it has units of "cases per person-time unit" and may assume *any* value greater than or equal to zero. By including time at risk in the definition, the incidence rate avoids the limitations of the cumulative incidence measure: The length of the observation period is automatically taken into account, and individuals entering or exiting the population because of migration, competing mortality, or any other reason are automatically accounted for. It may not always be practical, however, to calculate the time at risk for each individual in the population. A useful approximation to the time at risk can be obtained by multiplying the average of the population size at the beginning, middle, and end of the observation period by the length of time in the period (Lilienfeld, 1976).

Prevalence (P) depends on the incidence rate (I) and the average duration (D) of the disease. In a stable situation, the relationship may be expressed as:

$$P/(1 - P) = I \times D$$

Note that the denominator $(1 - P)$ is the proportion of the population that is "free of disease" and therefore at risk of getting it. The expression $P/(1 - P)$ is in the form of a statement of *odds*, i.e., the ratio of the probability of occurrence to the probability of nonoccurrence of disease, and is known as the *prevalence odds*. If the disease is very rare, i.e., P is very low, the prevalence odds approaches the prevalence, so the following approximation may be used:

$$P = I \times D$$

Cumulative incidence (CI) depends on the incidence rate (I) and the period at risk (t). It also depends on the number of individuals dying of causes other than the disease being studied, as previously mentioned. If this mortality from other diseases is disregarded, the relationship becomes:

$$CI = 1 - e^{(-I \times t)}$$

where e = 2.718 . . . is the base of the natural logarithms. Note that, for diseases with very low incidence rate or when the period is short, the following approximation may be used:

$$CI = I \times t$$

In epidemiologic studies, the frequency of disease occurrence among individuals who have a certain characteristic (called the *exposed group*) is generally compared with the corresponding frequency among those who do not have that characteristic (called the *unexposed group*). The compared groups are referred to as "exposed" and "unexposed" regardless of what the chosen characteristic is (i.e., it may be heredity or socioeconomic status). This is the fundamental way of studying the association between exposure and disease occurrence. The strength of the association must be described in order to assess whether or not an association may be causal. Comparisons of disease occurrence between exposed and unexposed groups involve one of the three measures of occurrence described already (P, CI, I). Absolute comparisons of these are based on the *difference* in occurrence of disease between exposed and unexposed groups, whereas relative comparisons are based on the *ratio* of occurrence of disease in exposed and unexposed groups. Relative comparisons of disease occurrence are more commonly used than absolute comparisons, since the importance of a difference in disease occurrence between two populations may not be meaningfully interpreted unless related to some baseline level of occurrence.

The *relative risk* or *risk ratio (RR)* is the ratio of the risk (i.e., the rate) of disease occurrence in exposed versus unexposed groups. It is called the *incidence rate ratio* when the incidence rate is the measure of occurrence used. If the period at risk is short, relative comparisons of cumulative incidence give approximately the same results as do relative comparisons of incidence rates, but as the observation period increases, the ratio of any two cumulative incidence measures approaches 1, whereas the incidence rate ratio is unaffected. If the prevalence is low and the duration of the disease (D) is the same among exposed and unexposed, relative comparisons of prevalence give approximately the same results as relative comparisons of incidence rates, but just as with CI, as the prevalence increases, prevalence ratios approach 1. However, if the prevalence odds is used in place of the prevalence, the resulting relative comparison, the *prevalence odds ratio,* is equivalent to the incidence rate ratio as long as D is constant:

$$\frac{P_1/(1-P_1)}{P_0/(1-P_0)} = \frac{I_1 D}{I_0 D} = \frac{I_1}{I_0}$$

where the subscripts are 1 for exposed and 0 for unexposed.

CAUSAL INFERENCE IN EPIDEMIOLOGIC STUDIES

The concept of *cause*, in its more general terms, is a deep subject in the philosophy of science far beyond the scope of this chapter, but intuitively, when two or more phenomena occur in a regular sequence dependably, we infer cause and effect. In epidemiology, the ultimate goal of causal inference is to explain and prevent the occurrence of disease. Characteristics (C) of individuals or their environments are said to be *associated* with disease (D) when C and D *covary*, that is, occur together more often than would be expected on the basis of chance alone. Reports of apparent covariation between C and D can have at least five possible explanations:

1. Random variation in both C and D.
2. Inaccurate methodology on the part of the investigator.
3. D is a cause of C.
4. Both C and D have a common cause X.
5. C is a cause of D.

Proper study design should eliminate explanations 1 and 2. If C occurs prior to D, then C is a *risk indicator* (or *risk factor*) for D and explanation 3 is eliminated. Note that risk indicators may be any demographic variable: age, gender, residence, occupation, smoking, etc. They may be useful in targeting high-risk groups for preventive efforts, a process known as *risk selection* or *risk assessment*, in which laboratory testing can play a major part (Iezzoni, 1997). Much effort in the design, conduct, and interpretation of epidemiologic studies must be directed toward distinguishing between explanation 4, the confounding explanation, in which C, although an indicator of risk, is a *confounder* (or *confounding variable*) to a true causal explanation of D. If explanation 5 is true and the association between C and D is causal, the incidence of D will be lower in the absence than in the presence of C.

To the extent that an observed association is strong enough to be regarded as causal, it becomes meaningful to discuss the magnitude in the reduction of disease occurrence that would result if the incidence rate in the exposed group were reduced to that of the unexposed group, i.e., the portion of the morbidity that is attributable to the exposure being studied. The *attributable proportion, AP* (also called attributable risk percent, attributable fraction, or etiologic fraction), is defined as:

$$AP = \frac{(RR - 1) \times f}{RR}$$

where RR is the rate ratio or "relative risk" (ratio of risk of occurrence in exposed and unexposed groups) and f is the proportion of those developing the disease who are exposed. Note that it is calculations of the attributable proportion that lead to commonly encountered statements such as that "80% of cancers are environmentally caused."

Generally, a disease has more than one cause, and often, one cause can contribute to the occurrence of more than one disease. Causes can be *direct* or *indirect* (i.e., activate other causes), and typically have degrees of directness that can be mapped in a *web of causation* for the disease being studied. Such a web may involve causes at different levels of organization from social to molecular and may reflect timeframes varying from multiple generations to milliseconds. A *sufficient cause* is one that inevitably brings certain consequences. Single causes are very seldom sufficient causes of disease. The vast majority of causes are not by themselves sufficient and are known as *contributing causes*. A *necessary cause* is one that must be present for the disease to occur. A cause may be necessary but not sufficient to cause disease. An example might be an infectious organism that is necessary for an infection but, in the absence of the appropriate conditions in the host, may be insufficient to do so.

Several contributing causes together typically form a sufficient cause, and one disease can have several sufficient causes, each of which may have one or more contributing causes in common. A contributing cause that is an element in all the sufficient causes is a necessary cause. As a practical matter, it is important to realize that knowledge of all contributing causes is not required in order to prevent disease. For example, by eliminating one of the contributors to one sufficient cause, all cases of the disease that result from this sufficient cause will be prevented. Each single cause of disease has an associated attributable proportion (AP), which represents the proportion of all cases that would not have occurred if the cause had been eliminated. The sum of all APs for all sufficient causes of a disease is always equal to 100%. The AP of a contributing cause is equal to the sum of the APs of all the sufficient causes in which it is an element. For every disease, the sum of all APs for contributing causes is 100% or more (generally more). The extent to which a contributing cause participates in the development of a disease is dependent on the presence of the other contributors to the corresponding sufficient cause. For example, if contributing cause A were present in 50% of cases, but the combination B + C + D only among 2%, then A will lead to the disease in $(.50) \times (.02) = .01$, i.e., 1% of individuals. Similarly, if the probability of occurrence of two or more contributing causes included in the same sufficient cause is increased, the effect on disease occurrence will be greater than the sum of the effects of the same increase in contributing causes acting through different sufficient causes. This is called *synergism* of effect.

BASIC EPIDEMIOLOGICAL STUDY DESIGNS

Research design for epidemiologic studies differs fundamentally from that in experimental research (e.g., pharmaceutical trials), in which the exposure is assigned to the study subjects by the investigator, often using randomized and/or blinded assignment. For both ethical and practical reasons this is usually impossible to do in epidemiological work, and these studies are based on naturally existing exposure conditions (Spilker, 1991). Two basic study designs are used in epidemiological research to compare incidence rates between exposed and unexposed groups, *cohort* (or "follow-up") and *case-control* (or "cross-sectional") studies. In the cohort type of study design, all study subjects are assigned an exposure category at the start of the study. The categories may be dichotomous (exposed/unexposed) or multiple (unexposed, low exposure, high exposure). All subjects are then followed up for a defined period of time, and all new cases of the disease or condition occurring in the exposed and unexposed groups are identified. This is called a *prospective* study design. The product of the population size and the time period at risk (i.e., person-time observed) is referred to as the *study base* from which the cases arise. The measures of occurrence for the exposed and unexposed groups are determined and compared in either an absolute or relative fashion.

The selection of the unexposed group is a critical aspect of the cohort study design. The unexposed group is intended to provide information about the disease incidence rate that would be expected in the exposed group if the exposure under study did not affect the occurrence of the disease. Therefore, it should be selected in such a way that it is similar to the exposed group with regard to other risk indicators for the disease under study. There are three main approaches to defining the unexposed group. With an *internal comparison*, a single cohort is identified that contains a sufficient number of exposed and unexposed subjects, whereas with an *external comparison*, an exposed cohort is identified and efforts are made to find another cohort that is unexposed but is similar in other respects to the exposed cohort. With the third approach, *comparison with the "general" population*, an exposed cohort is identified and comparisons are made with the disease incidence in, for example, the total population of a defined geographic region (considered as "unexposed").

There are several drawbacks to using the general population as a comparison group in cohort studies. The *"healthy worker effect"* is a bias that results because subjects who are employed in certain occupations are healthy enough to work and therefore at lower risk of developing many diseases. This effect could lead to underestimation of the relative morbidity in the exposed group. The *dilution* effect occurs when the total population is used to represent the "unexposed" group, and exposed individuals are included among the "unexposed." Unless the proportion of exposed individuals in the population is low, this will result in underestimation of the relative morbidity in the exposed group. *Differential case-finding* occurs when certain screening procedures are used to a greater extent in the exposed group than in the unexposed group, leading to more complete case identification in the exposed group. Note that confounding may occur if a risk indicator other than the studied exposure is unequally distributed between the groups. If recognized, this can be corrected in the data analysis by standardization. It may be necessary to select exposed and unexposed groups with similar distributions of geographic area, ethnicity, and socioeconomic status and to follow them during the same observation period to avoid these problems. Selecting more than one unexposed group can reveal to what extent the study results are influenced by the selection of an unexposed group (a procedure known as *sensitivity analysis*). Separate analyses using these groups that yield similar results indicate that the results probably were not influenced by the choice of the unexposed group, i.e., were *robust*. Another check on the comparability between the exposed and the unexposed group is to include comparisons of the occurrence of diseases that are not expected to be associated with the exposure under study.

Retrospective cohort studies are based on information about exposure and disease collected in the past. For instance, a cancer registry or cause-of-death registry may be used as a source of information about cases, with considerable savings in the cost of case finding. Note that the accuracy of such a study depends upon the completeness of disease ascertainment in the registry for the population and time period under study. Similarly, information on "exposure" may be obtained from census data or registries providing information on certain occupational groups. The savings may be substantial, but the quality of exposure information should be examined before relying on such a source. In addition, information on relevant confounders may not be available from these sources.

In *case-control studies*, information is obtained on all *cases* that occur in the study population during a defined observation period. In addition, a comparison group of "*controls*" is selected as a representative sample of the study population. Ideally the control group reflects the exposure distribution in the entire study population. Exposure information is then obtained for cases and controls only, rather than for all members of the population. There are two basic approaches to control selection. Utilizing a *random sample* of the study population has the advantage that the controls will be representative of the study population in a formal (statistical) sense and therefore the selection process for controls does not introduce any systematic error. This option obviously requires that the population be accessible for random sampling. Potential disadvantages of random sampling for control selection are the possibility of a high nonresponse rate among healthy population controls, and the possibility of differences in the quality of exposure information between cases and healthy controls.

Utilizing a sample of the study population that is not randomly selected is the only option when the cases are identified in such a way that the study population is not accessible for random sampling. For example, if the cases are patients diagnosed with the disease being studied in a particular clinic, these patients most likely do not represent all cases of the disease occurring in a population from which a random sample may be drawn, and therefore a nonrandom selection of controls is necessary. Sometimes this approach is used for other reasons, such as reducing nonresponse among controls or improving the comparability of exposure information between cases and controls. Controls may be selected, for example, from patients who have been *hospitalized (hospital controls)* or who have died (*dead controls*) during the observation period from diseases other than the one under study. While such nonrandom selection schemes may result in greater comparability of cases and controls, controls selected in this way may not reflect the exposure distribution in the overall study population, thus possibly introducing a systematic error. In case-control studies, controls are sometimes selected by individual *matching* to the cases: For every case, one or more controls are selected who are similar to that case in certain respects. Cases and controls are matched on potential confounders, such as age, sex, and residence, for which information can be obtained before data collection begins. The implications of matching in case-control studies are complex. Matching is performed for the purpose of reducing random error, not confounding. Matching can actually introduce problems, since each case and its corresponding control must be kept together during analysis.

There are advantages and disadvantages of both the cohort and case-control designs. Cohort studies have a simple, logical structure that leads to measurements of disease incidence for the exposed and unexposed groups, or each category of exposure, if several are used. This design permits absolute as well as relative comparisons of disease incidence among the exposed and unexposed groups. When the induction period (time between exposure and disease appearance for the disease under study) is long, one or more decades may have to elapse between exposure and the beginning of the study observation period. This delay can often be avoided by collecting exposure information retrospectively in cohort studies as well as in case-control studies.

Case-control studies, like cohort studies, are based on follow-up of incident cases in a certain study population during a defined observation period. Case-control studies, however, use exposure information from a sample of the study population rather than from the whole study population. Unless the disease incidence is very high, obtaining exposure information for a sample of the study population will be much less expensive and can yield more information on exposure, as fewer subjects need to be studied. The case-control design therefore makes investigations based on large study populations more feasible, an important consideration since large studies are usually needed to reduce random error.

A major disadvantage of the case-control design is the difficulty in selecting a satisfactory control group, with the consequent problem of introducing systematic error into the study by the selection of controls. When the control group is defined as a random sample of the study population, control selection is a simple technical procedure and introduces no systematic error beyond what would be present in a cohort study using the entire study population. Using information from a sample (controls) rather than from the entire study population does increase random variability, but when the size of the control group is adequate, this effect is small or negligible. The amount of random error that can be removed by expanding the control group to include the entire study population is often trivial, whereas the corresponding cost would be great. In case-control studies involving contact with study subjects or their relatives, the study subjects usually answer questions about previous exposure only after the cases have fallen ill. The cases, therefore, may have spent more time thinking about past exposures and causes of their disease, while the controls have no motivation to do so. This difference between cases and controls in the accuracy and completeness of exposure information can introduce a *"recall bias"* into the study. A similar bias may be seen in cohort studies in which, for some reason, exposure information is obtained only after the cases have been identified.

ADJUSTING AND COMPARING DATA SETS

Crude measures of disease occurrence (e.g., crude prevalence, and crude incidence rate) are calculated for the general population as a whole. *Specific measures* of disease occurrence (e.g., age-specific prevalence, etc.) are calculated separately for parts of the population (called *"strata"*) when there is reason to believe that disease occurrence varies from one of these subgroups to another. These variations may remain hidden if only crude measures are used. *Stratification* is one way to study and control for the effects of variables other than exposure and disease in the data analysis. Stratification by gender, residence, or age, for example, means that the data are divided into categories of male/female, urban/rural, or into categories of age. *Confounding* occurs when some cause other than the exposure under study is more or less prevalent in the exposed group than in the unexposed group. When levels of the confounding factor stratify data, for example in male versus female gender, each stratum will be free from confounding by the stratification variable. That is, if the association between exposure and disease is analyzed separately in males and females, each of the two strata will give an estimate of the exposure, free of confounding by gender. Often these stratum-specific results are not reported separately, but are pooled into a single result.

Effect modification in a stratified analysis means that the effect of the exposure is stronger in some strata than in others. It is present when the relative risk relating exposure and disease is greater in one stratum than in another. If, for example, the relative risk (ratio of the incidence rate among exposed to that among unexposed) were 2.5 among indoor workers and 3.4 among outdoor workers, work location would modify the effect of exposure and thus be an effect modifier. *Risk adjustment* or *standardization of rates* is a type of stratification in which correction is made for the possibility that a potentially relevant characteristic, such as age or serum cholesterol level, is differentially distributed among strata. The comparison of two populations based on comparing crude disease rates may not be valid if their members differ significantly in the distribution of some potentially relevant characteristic. The magnitude of a crude measure for a population depends not only on the magnitude of the specific measures that apply to subgroups of the population, but also on the way the population is distributed over the different subgroups. The crude rate is a weighted average of the stratum-specific rates, with weights proportional to the number of individuals or person-years in each stratum.

Adjustment may be direct or indirect. With *direct adjustment* (for example, on age), crude population rates for each stratum are recalculated to what they would have been had the age distributions in both strata been equal to that in a standard population. An example of such a standard population might be the combined exposed and unexposed populations being compared. Thus the age-specific rates (crude rate for each age stratum treated separately) would be multiplied by the following proportion:

$$\frac{\text{Stratum-specific number of exposed individuals} + \text{unexposed individuals}}{\text{Total number of individuals exposed and unexposed}}$$

to give *age-adjusted strata*. All such strata in each population would then be summed to give the *age-adjusted rate* for that population. Then finally, taking the difference or ratio of these age-adjusted rates for the two populations gives an absolute or relative age-adjusted comparison between them—for example, the *standardized incidence rate ratio (SRR)* is the ratio of age-adjusted incidence rates between two populations. The limitation of adjustment is the choice of standard population. In principle, the standard population should reflect the distribution of the population for which effects are to be estimated, but it may not be clear what this means. In the preceding example, a different adjusted relative risk would have resulted if a different standard population had been chosen.

In many real examples, such as those often found in hospital-based studies, the numbers of individuals in each stratum of the exposed population may be so small that direct comparisons are not meaningful. In such cases, the comparison can be made between the observed number of cases in the exposed population (A) and the corresponding expected number (E). E is the number of cases that would have occurred in the exposed population had all the stratum-specific incidence rates in the exposed population been the same as those in the unexposed population. Multiplying each stratum by the ratio A/E, a process called *indirect adjustment*, is therefore equivalent to standardizing the incidence rates in the exposed and unexposed populations, with the unexposed population now serving as the standard population. This ratio A/E is expressed as a percentage, called the *standardized morbidity (or mortality) ratio (SMR)*.

COMPARISONS OF EPIDEMIOLOGIC DATA SETS

The evaluation of the relative accuracy of epidemiologic studies has two aspects: validity and precision. *Validity* is the degree to which the study measures what it is intended to measure. Lack of validity is referred to as *bias* or systematic error. Systematic errors, leading to low validity, can arise in several different ways. *Biases to internal validity* are factors that cause the observed results of a study to not accurately reflect the effect of exposure under the circumstances of investigation. They include the following types of confounders: *Patient selection bias* occurs when subjects in the exposed group differ from those in the control group in a way that can affect the outcomes. With *contamination bias,* subjects presumed to be unexposed are actually exposed, whereas with *dilution bias,* subjects presumed to be exposed are actually not exposed (Michael et al., 1984).

Errors in the measurement of outcomes may occur in a number of ways. For example, this may occur when databases established for one purpose (e.g., paying claims) are used for another (e.g., estimating outcomes). It may also occur when the interests and study focus of the investigator change after the data elements of the database have been determined. It may occur when the outcome is determined by a test that is not "gold standard" or when the gold standard changes through the introduction of new technology, or in situations where interobserver variability is significant. *Ascertainment bias* may occur in retrospective studies due to loss of records or inaccuracies of memory. *Loss to follow-up* may occur in those cases in which the lost individuals differ as a group from the group as a whole. It is important to bear in mind that multiple and nested biases can and do occur. Any combination of these biases to internal validity can coexist within a study.

Biases to external validity and comparability between studies arise when the circumstances of the study differ from the circumstances of interest in ways that affect the outcome of interest. These situations include the following: *Population bias* occurs when differences exist between the individuals in the circumstances of investigation and the individuals in the circumstances of interest, including differences of age, gender, concurrent disease, treatment compliance, etc. With *intensity bias,* differences exist in the delivery of exposure or interventions between the circumstances of the study and those of interest, including differences of intervention (dose, frequency, technique, and equipment) provider (skill, training), or setting (inpatient vs. outpatient). Differences may also exist in the length of time individuals are followed. This *length of follow-up bias* differs in importance depending on the measure of effect chosen.

The propensity of different study designs to biases is shown in the following table:

Study design	Patient selection bias	Dilution/ contamination bias	Outcome error	Ascertainment bias	Population bias	Intensity bias
Case-control	+ +	0	+	+ + +	0	0
Cohort	+	+ +	+	0	+	+

Precision is the reproducibility of a study result, that is, the degree of resemblance among study results, were the study to be repeated under similar circumstances. Lack of precision is referred to as *random error*. Reports of properly conducted epidemiologic studies should always state an estimate of the precision of the basic measures of disease occurrence (P, CI, I). The observed measure should be reported along with a confidence interval that provides some information as to the precision of the observed value. A confidence interval of 95%, say, is a range of values constructed to account for random variation in such a way that, if there were no systematic errors in the study, the probability that the interval would contain the true value is 95%. This means that, on the average, 95% of such intervals from valid studies would contain the true parameter value and 5% would fail to do so. Thus, by assessing the confidence interval, information about the precision of the study is obtained. This assessment can be of great importance in epidemiologic studies where random variation stemming from a small number of diseased subjects plays an important role in interpretation. To calculate the confidence interval a probability model is needed. The models used for this purpose are described in the references (e.g., Ahlbom and Norell, 1990).

STATISTICAL CONSIDERATIONS IN EPIDEMIOLOGICAL STUDIES

The purpose of a *significance test* is to determine the degree of consistency between a specific *hypothesis H* and a set of data. In most cases, H is a simple description of some aspect of a particular population and the collected data are obtained from a sample drawn from the population. While the sample is thought to be representative of the population, it is clear that a different sample would give rise to a different set of data. If the observed results are inconsistent with H, then either (1) H is true and imprecision or random error accounts for the observed results, or (2) H is false and the difference between the true situation and H is the reason for the observed results

A significance test assumes that a specific *null hypothesis H_0* about a population (e.g., that there is no difference between exposed and unexposed groups) is true and compares the outcome observed in a sample of the population with all other possible outcomes that sampling uncertainty might have generated. In general terms, six elements must necessarily be present to carry out a test of significance properly:

(1) an explicit statement of H_0, (2) data representing a random sample of the population, (3) a full set of comparable events to the outcome, (4) the probability distribution of the test statistic, (5) the rank order of all possible outcomes, and (6) a valid formula for calculating significance level.

Examples of *standard tests of significance* devised by statisticians that specify these elements include: Fisher's test for 2×2 contingency tables, Chi square test for 2×2 tables, the *F*-test, and Student's *t*-tests. Consult standard references in biostatistics for the specific proper use of these tests (e.g., Matthews and Farewell, 1985). The *confidence interval* on a parameter describing a set of data identifies the set of all the parameter's values that are consistent with the observed data. It includes every possible value of the parameter, which, if tested as a specific null hypothesis in the usual way, would not lead to the conclusion that the data contradict that particular null hypothesis.

Sample size (N) is often a critical consideration in the design and interpretation of epidemiologic studies. Studies involving small N may not be worth doing. Reasons to maximize N include ensuring the effectiveness of randomization, minimizing the problem of multiple comparisons, and maximizing the expected value of true positive conclusions. *Randomization* is undertaken in studies in order to try to ensure that any important factor that has been overlooked, inadvertently or unconsciously, during study design, has an effect that is roughly similar in all exposure groups. The effectiveness of randomization, however, depends on total sample size. So randomizing a large number of participants is more likely to achieve the intended result. *Multiple comparisons* arise in the context of stratified analyses. If a study involves only a few participants, there will be little possibility of doing a stratified analysis, since each stratum is likely to contain too few subjects to allow statistically significant comparisons. Large studies make stratification more feasible and meaningful.

For these reasons, it is essential that a calculation of the required sample size be part of the design of all epidemiologic studies. *Sample size calculations* are always approximate, since it is impossible to predict the exact outcome of any particular study in advance. Moreover, sample size calculations are frequently complicated. Nonetheless, their importance is demonstrated by the fact that they provide information about two critical study design questions:

1. How many subjects should be involved?
2. Is the study worth doing if only n subjects (a fixed number) participate?

The answers to these questions enable an investigator to evaluate a study proposal critically and to decide whether or not to proceed as planned, given the available resources of personnel, funds, and participants. The particular calculations of sample size used depend on the primary question the researchers want to investigate and the way in which it is to be answered.

Suppose, for example, that a cohort study of an environmental exposure is being planned. The chief purpose of the study is to compare one or more specific health outcomes in exposed versus unexposed individuals. The answer to this primary question, let us say, can be expressed in terms of a clinically relevant difference in incidence rates. The study is being conducted to determine the degree to which the results are consistent with the null hypothesis H_0 of no difference in incidence rates. Either such a difference will be demonstrated, or the data will be judged consistent with the null hypothesis. It is conventional at the study design phase to assume that failure to reject the null hypothesis is equivalent to concluding that the null hypothesis is true. (It must be noted that this convention, while convenient at the study design stage, is inappropriate at the final stage of data analysis.) The true situation in the study population concerning the null hypothesis can never be known for certain. Also, with respect to the true situation, the researcher's final conclusions regarding the incidence rate difference may be correct or wrong. The situation then, may be summarized in a fourfold table of correct and erroneous conclusions, thus:

	Investigator's conclusion that H_0 is true	Investigator's conclusion that H_0 is false
Actual situation that H_0 is true	Correct conclusion	False positive conclusion (Type I error)
Actual situation that H_0 is false	False negative conclusion (Type II error)	Correct conclusion

The probabilities of correct and erroneous conclusions are as follows:

	Investigator's conclusion that H_0 is true	Investigator's conclusion that H_0 is false
Actual situation that H_0 is true	$1 - \alpha$	α
Actual situation that H_0 is false	β	$1 - \beta$

Since α and β both represent probabilities of making an erroneous decision, ideally they should be close to zero. Unfortunately, if α is decreased without changing the total sample size N, then β necessarily increases. Conversely, if β must decrease without changing N, then α necessarily increases. Only by increasing N can α and β both be simultaneously reduced. If no exposure difference exists, then α is simply the probability of obtaining an unlikely outcome in that situation and wrongly deciding that the data contradict the null hypothesis. This probability is precisely the significance level of the data with respect to H_0, i.e., the p-value for statistical significance. The value of α that the investigator uses to conclude whether H_0 is true or false is usually regarded as fixed in advance. In this case, p will decrease as the total sample size increases. The decision regarding an adequate sample size for a given study will necessarily be a compromise, balancing what can be achieved statistically with a sample size that is practical.

If a real exposure difference exists, i.e., if H_0 is false, the probability that the investigator will correctly conclude that this is so is $(1 - \beta)$. This probability depends largely on N, the total sample size and on the actual magnitude of the exposure difference (δ). The reason for the dependence on sample size is fairly simple. A larger sample contains more information about characteristics that are of interest, and therefore allows more precise estimation of the true situation in the study population. Therefore by increasing sample size, we increase the ability to detect any real exposure difference that exists. This increased ability to determine whether H_0 is true or false is translated into an increased probability, $(1 - \beta)$, that a correct conclusion will be reached when H_0 is false. Since $(1 - \beta) + \beta = 1$, if $(1 - \beta)$ increases, then the false negative probability β necessarily decreases. Therefore increasing N can also be viewed as a means of decreasing the false negative rate when a real exposure difference exists.

The probability $(1 - \alpha)$ of detecting a specified real exposure difference, δ, is called the statistical *power* of the study. A powerful study is one with a high probability of detecting an important exposure difference. The ratio of expected false positive (α) to expected true positive conclusions or power $(1 - \alpha)$ is usually fixed at the study design stage, and power decreases with decreasing N. Therefore, attempting to combine conclusions from an increased number of small studies increases the likelihood that any positive conclusions will be false compared with the conclusions of a smaller number of large studies.

We are now in a position to state, in precise terms, the two questions about any study that sample size calculations will answer: (1) If the probability of a false positive conclusion is fixed at α, what total sample size N is required to ensure that the probability of detecting a clinically relevant difference of a given magnitude δ is $(1 - \beta)$? (2) If the probability of a false positive conclusion is fixed at α and a specific sample size N is employed, what is the probability, $(1 - \beta)$, that the study will detect a clinically relevant difference of a given magnitude δ, i.e., what is the power of the study under these conditions?

Note that the answer to either question is not a single number, but rather a table or graph of sample sizes, N, or probabilities, $(1 - \beta)$, for different possible triplet combinations of values for α, δ, and $(1 - \beta)$ in the first case, or α, δ, and N in the second. Tables for sample size and power calculations are available in reference books such as Fleiss (1973).

Other considerations in the determination of adequate sample size include the relative sizes of the exposed and unexposed groups, possible dropout rates in these groups, and lack of uniform standards in evaluating patient characteristics or outcomes (called *differential case-finding*).

COMBINING EPIDEMIOLOGIC DATA SETS

The estimation problem is one of the most important and difficult problems in science. The synthesis of evidence to estimate the outcomes of different actions or occurrences is the basis for our understanding of disease. Ideally, for every question there should be a collection of studies that point directly to the answer, but this is rarely the case in reality, due to a variety of practical problems, such as (1) multiple pieces of evidence to be synthesized, (2) different experimental designs in the different pieces of evidence (e.g., clinical series, randomized controlled trials), (3) different types of outcomes (e.g., dichotomous. or continuous), (4) different measures of effect: study results expressed as outcomes, relative risks, odds ratios, etc., (5) biases to internal validity, external validity, and comparability, (6) indirect evidence: studies may provide evidence about intermediate outcomes (e.g., serum cholesterol level) rather than the health outcome of ultimate interest (e.g., probability of myocardial infarction), (7) mixed comparisons—when there are several exposures or interventions of interest, available evidence can compare different pairs of interventions, e.g., one study might compare treatment or exposure A with B, another B with C, and to determine the effect of A versus C, it is necessary to synthesize these mixed comparisons, and (8) gaps in experimental evidence often leave no option but to use informal evidence interpreted subjectively.

The most common approach to the estimation problem is *global subjective judgment*. The people making the judgments gather all the evidence they want to consider, mix it in their heads, and develop an impression of the outcome of interest. The result is an opinion (judgment) based on perceptions (subjective) that attempts to capture all the evidence, all the factors, and all the biases, all at once (global). The problems with this approach include: (1) Real-world problems can be too complex for it to work, (2) different people can arrive at very different judgments, (3) the process is closed to review, and (4) there is no way to tell if the answer arrived at in this way is wrong.

Objective approaches to the estimation problem include a set of sophisticated quantitative statistical methods known collectively as *meta-analysis*. These methods provide explicit objective ways to utilize multiple studies to structure a problem, break it into parts, focus attention on one part at a time, perform calculations, reconstruct the parts, present a solution, and allow concurrent review and interpretation by others. The first step in conducting a meta-analysis is to focus the question or questions to be answered by the analysis. The following are examples of the basic logical sequences from interventions to outcomes that are presented by different types of population-based studies in the literature that should provide guidance in this area:

Preventive interventions:

Intervention → Change probability of disease → change outcomes *or*
Intervention → change behavior → change probability of disease → change outcomes

Diagnostic interventions:

Intervention → diagnose disease → institute/change treatment → change outcomes

The next step is to develop a search strategy for retrieving literature on the topic of interest. It should be explicit and reproducible; e.g., a MedLine or Grateful Med search utilizing title key words is appropriate.

After the papers have been collected and examined, it is very helpful to summarize them in the form of an *evidence table* that includes such information as:

The type of design (e.g., randomized controlled trial, case-control study).

The number of individuals involved (e.g., number of people in the control and treated groups of a randomized controlled trial, the number of cases and controls in a case-control study).

The outcomes measured (e.g., heart attacks after one year).

The types of individuals (e.g., men age 60 to 70, with an acute myocardial infarction within the past 6 months).

The interventions compared (e.g., aspirin vs. chicken soup).

Any biases to internal validity, along with estimates of their magnitude, either discussed by the investigators or suspected by the meta-analyst.

Any biases to external validity relative to the comparison of interest to the meta-analyst (e.g., year in which the study was conducted, technique of the intervention).

Any other factors that might affect interpretation (e.g., length of follow-up).

The observed outcomes of the study (e.g., number of heart attacks in the control and treated groups).

The reported effect of the intervention (e.g., point estimates and confidence limits of the percent reduction in probability of a heart attack).

Finally, combine the data sets by the *data pooling* method if appropriate, or by using one of the specialized statistical procedures developed for meta-analysis known as the effect size, variance weighting, Mantel–Haenszel, Peto, Der Simonian and Laird, or confidence profile methods as described by Eddy et al. (1992). Pooling can be used when the parameter of interest is a rate and the studies being analyzed all provide data in a form that can be used as numerator and denominator for computing this rate. All the numerators are added, all the denominators are added, and their pooled rate (weighted average) is calculated by dividing the sum of the numerators by the sum of the denominators. This method, though seemingly straightforward, requires the assumption of strict identity in the circumstances of investigation of all the studies regarding any factors that could affect the rates (i.e., requires the assumption that they are all controlled by and reflect the same underlying true rate). With the same stringent requirements, the data pooling approach can also be applied to the meta-analysis of controlled trials. In this case, weighted averages for the rates are calculated for the treated and control groups separately, and as long as the treated groups are similar for all the studies, and the control groups are similar for all studies, the results can be compared to estimate the treatment effect.

In contrast to data pooling, with its simplicity, but severe restrictions, the general and powerful *confidence profile* method of meta-analysis deals with the estimation problem as a problem in decision-making. The first step is to evaluate evidence to estimate the information on which the decision will be based (the parameters of interest). Then follows a series of value judgments in which the parameters of interest are weighed, and the option expected to have the most desirable outcomes is chosen. Available in the form of software program (*FAST*PRO,* ©Academic Press), the method can be employed in either a Bayesian or non-Bayesian fashion to synthesize an unlimited number of pieces of evidence. It can be used to analyze any of eight basic types of study design: clinical series (one-arm prospective trial), randomized controlled trials (two-arm prospective), m-arm prospective, multidose prospective, 2×2 case-control studies (retrospective), $2 \times k$ retrospective (case-control studies with exposures of different intensities), continuous dose retrospective, and cross-sectional. It can be used to analyze studies involving outcomes that are dichotomous (e.g., survive/not survive), continuous (e.g., degree of weight loss, IQ), categorical (e.g., cancer stage), or count (e.g., number of anginal attacks per week).

The confidence profile method can also be used to estimate the effect of an exposure/intervention compared with an alternative in terms of absolute differences, relative differences (e.g., percent change), ratios (e.g., relative risk), odds ratios, and effect size. It can synthesize evidence from different studies with different effect measures, including converting effect measures to forms that are more useful in decision making (e.g., converting an odds ratio into a difference in probabilities). It can adjust for biases to internal validity, including dilution, contamination, errors in outcome measures, errors in attribution of exposure to intervention, patient selection bias, differences in providers, settings, and follow-up care. It can accommodate compound and nested biases and incorporate uncertainty about magnitudes of any or all biases through the use of probability distributions, and it can adjust for population bias, intensity bias, and differences in follow-up times between studies.

The confidence profile method is potentially useful as a guide to new directions in research. It can link an unlimited number of pieces of indirect evidence into a chain. It can relate exposures/interventions that are not directly compared in any studies, provided only that existing studies relate pairs of other interventions that eventually link the intervention of interest to the alternative of interest. It can accommodate the use of subjective judgments ("clinical judgment") if necessary. It allows sensitivity analysis of how changes in any one parameter will change any other parameter. It can use the results of a previous analysis to calculate the statistical power of a new experiment, and thus to estimate information useful for determining the value of conducting additional research on any parameter. It can estimate the probability that a new experiment will deliver results within any specified range. It can estimate the mean and variance of a new parameter distribution that incorporates a proposed experiment, use information on covariance to determine how changes in mean and variance of any one parameter will change the estimated mean and variance of any other parameter.

REFERENCES

Ahlbom A, Norell S. *Introduction to Modern Epidemiology*. Epidemiology Resources, Inc., Newton Lower Falls, MA, 1990.

Eddy DM, Hasselblad V, Schachter R. *Meta-Analysis by the Confidence Profile Method*. Academic Press, Boston, 1992.

Fleiss JL. *Statistical Methods for Rates and Proportions*. Wiley Interscience, New York, 1973.

Friedman GD. *Primer of Epidemiology*, third edition. McGraw-Hill, New York, 1987.

Hedges LV, Olkin I. *Statistical Methods for Meta-Analysis*. Academic Press, New York, 1985.

Iezzoni LI (ed.). *Risk Adjustment for Measuring Healthcare Outcomes*, second edition. Health Administration Press, Chicago, 1997.

Last JM, Wallace RB, et al. (eds.). *Maxcy-Rosenau-Last Public Health & Preventive Medicine*, 13th edition. Appleton & Lange, Norwalk, CT, 1992.

Lilienfeld AM. *Foundations of Epidemiology*. Oxford University Press, New York, 1976.

Matthews DE, Farewell V. *Using and Understanding Medical Statistics*. S. Karger, Basel, 1985.

Michael M, Boyce WT, Wilcox AJ. *Biomedical Bestiary: An Epidemiologic Guide to Flaws and Fallacies in the Medical Literature*. Little, Brown, Boston, 1984.

Spilker B. *Guide to Clinical Trials*. Raven Press, New York, 1991.

Chapter 5

Outcomes Measurement: Collecting Valid and Reliable Information Using Surveys

K. M. Peddecord, L. K. Hofherr, and D. Francis

OVERVIEW: NOT AN "ALL-IN-ONE" CHAPTER BUT A "READER'S GUIDE"

It would be presumptuous or naïve to believe this chapter could include a significant proportion of what you need to know to conduct a valid and cost-effective survey. Rather than an "everything you need to know" chapter, our goal is to provide a guide. We have striven to provide a useful framework and a guide to the critical issues and steps in collecting high-quality information. Our selection of topics is based on our experiences as teachers and researchers, and we have cited texts and publications that are useful resources. Survey research on laboratory outcomes issues is limited, but we anticipate that it will continue to grow in the future. While we do not intend this to be a literature review, we have also provided selected citations of successful surveys (Hofherr et al., 1993; Rau et al., 1996; Peddecord et al., 1993, 1996) that assess various aspects of laboratory management and laboratory associated outcomes.

Information gathered from surveys is increasingly important in a competitive market oriented health care system. The outcomes movement, with its increased emphasis on measurable results, is driven largely by purchasers' and patients' desire to understand the value they are purchasing for their increasing health-care insurance expenditures. Organizations that understand the needs and wants of their important customers are more likely to prosper. Surveys are the most important method of measuring patient- (or client-) based outcomes. Patient-based outcomes are defined as "results" that a patient can "understand" and report. Common outcomes that may "result," at least in part, from medical care include such things as reduction of pain, increased ability to complete activities of daily living, early return to school or work following illness, being treated professionally when having a blood test drawn, being able to trust their physician, satisfaction with the waiting time at their physician's office, or just plain feeling better. Quantitatively measuring all of these outcomes requires surveys.

PLANNING THE SURVEY: OBJECTIVES FOR THE STUDY

Designing a survey should be thought of as a process. Start by clarifying the reason for performing a survey. As with most planning, begin by thinking about the end. Invest a sufficient amount of time in the beginning in assessing what your products will be. Before designing your questionnaire, clearly determine what you want to do with the results. Always develop ideas that need an answer, then develop the questions to fill in these gaps. How will you utilize the information gathered? Is timing critical? Do you need to use the information to intervene on a regular basis or can it exist as a final report? How large a survey do you want to perform? Is it manageable? Can you get results back in time for your intervention? Is the length appropriate to the population and the methods of collection; i.e., is the survey more than 15 minutes or 2 to 3 pages?

Identifying objectives means moving beyond the vague questions. What is the satisfaction level of physicians who use our STAT lab? Move beyond the "outcomes" to the "why" of satisfaction or confidence in your services. Another method to help bring focus to your objectives (and eventually your survey instrument) is to create mock tables for your publication or final report. Moving back from the end is the same process used by an information systems analyst when designing a report from an information system. Knowing that we want to differentiate the levels of satisfaction between frequent and infrequent users of the laboratory assures that we will ask a question that categorizes physicians according to how frequently they order a specific service or have contact with the laboratory.[1]

PLANNING: FINDING RESOURCES

Planning is seldom a step-by-step sequential process; many tasks need to be done concurrently. One task that has to be done early in your planning is

---

[1]A cardinal rule in any customer survey is: Determine how familiar the respondents are with the product or service of interest. Do they know about the service or use it everyday? Respondents may have vastly different opinions about the quality of service based on how often they use the service. Does familiarity breed contentment or contempt? We may want to give much more importance to problems that are reported frequently by someone who **utilizes the laboratory often or who experiences laboratory services often** than those of a client who only occasionally uses its services.

that you will need a realistic assessment of resources. What resources are needed for the survey and what is the budget? Yes, the perfect survey can be planned, but finding the budget to support it is a challenge that needs to be confronted early in the planning. Do you have human resources? Are there staff or researchers in your organizations that can assist you? How much time and expertise can you, the principal investigator or leader of the survey team, devote? What is the depth of the team's expertise? Can you afford to hire a vendor? What part of the work should you "outsource" and still keep the survey on track? Where can you find advice?

Outsourcing is new jargon for contracting for a service from a vendor rather than doing the work "in-house." Contracting for various parts of the survey has advantages. Much of the work of a well-conducted survey, and other research for that matter, is tedious and requires significant record keeping. This includes critical tasks such as repeated telephoning to set appointments for a phone interview; sending out surveys to nonrespondents who lost your second survey; entering data into a database; calling a difficult-to-reach academician in a remote time zone who has a survey with answers you want; etc. Do you have reliable clerical staff that can be devoted to these tasks? Is there someone who can format and reformat your questionnaire to make it user-friendly? Deciding to outsource leads naturally to the next big concern, to whom do you give the work and what do they charge for their services? Several such sources are listed in the resource appendix.

INFORMATION IS A CONTINUOUS NEED: THINKING LONG TERM

Too often we think of collecting data using a survey as an extraordinary event. We collect our data from our customers or patients, we look at it, we do our report, and we put it aside until the next project. This is, unfortunately, how we often think of quality assurance. We get ready for our Joint Commission on Accreditation of Health care Organizations (JCAHO) or state inspections, we have the inspection, we accept our deficiencies, we learn, we write our plan for correction, and then we go back to our real job for the next two years. This approach isn't attuned with a philosophy of continuous quality improvement. While some outcome surveys may be one-time events, many outcome studies are ongoing or prospective follow-ups. We want to understand the health status at 6 months, 12 months, and 24 months. Surveys in the context of a quality improvement program are also continuous. We identify our performance level today, change the way we provide care, and reassess using a second survey to determine how customer satisfaction ratings or health status have changed. One quality improvement survey often leads to another (McLaughlin and Kaluzny, 1994).

Benchmarking. Another reason to view surveys as an ongoing activity is enhancing the usefulness of the information from a single survey. While a single survey can yield important information, this single value without a norm or benchmark has no comparative value. How do our patient's outcomes compare with the well-established health plan or the medical school teaching hospital? We won't know without comparative data. A popular term in today's measurement-driven health-care sectors is *benchmark*. When we have results from our survey, what do the numbers mean? Is 80% satisfaction good or poor? This is where large survey consultants and vendors have a distinct advantage. They have comparative data to help, at least in a relative way, to understand what the numbers mean. At a minimum, we at least need to how we have fared in the past.

SURVEY DESIGN: KEY ISSUES IN DESIGNING AND EXECUTING YOUR SURVEY

As with many other endeavors, systematic planning for a survey is critical to success of this data collection effort. Several survey research texts use the term "total survey process" (Backstrom and Hursh, 1963) to identify a comprehensive framework for managing the survey process. The theme of this approach is that information collection is a system and that the entire process must be properly managed in order to obtain maximum value from the resources expended on the survey. If several steps in the process are optimized while others are neglected, the entire system may be a failure. This notion of "system" is very much in keeping with the tenets of total quality management (McLaughlin and Kaluzny, 1994). In the laboratory literature, a systems approach to quality has been characterized as "the total testing process."

PROPER SAMPLING

Can we identify and contact the individuals or organizations that have information of value to our outcome study? Do we have the correct mailing list? If not, can we purchase or develop that list? Obtaining a list of medical staff of a hospital, or of medical groups, who are sharing risk in a managed care arrangement, is not difficult. On the other hand, finding a list of all the primary care physicians in a community who are treating 10 or more HIV-infected patients each month is a daunting challenge. Lists from professional organizations are often useful, but these "opportunity" or "convenience" samples may be highly biased. If the bias is that they are all interested in infectious disease, that may be just what you need. These physicians will be the most knowledgeable and the most interested in responding to a survey. However, if you want to make estimates about treatment patterns in the community as a whole, the list is both biased and inappropriate for the intended purpose.[2] Again, focusing on the objective of the survey should guide you to the type of mailing or telephone list that will be the best suited for your project. No matter the source of the list, it should have demographics of everyone in the sample to whom you mail the survey or plan to contact by telephone to survey. Collecting demographics from the respondents will enable you to do a basic comparison of how the responders compare to the entire population from which the sample was taken.

HUMAN SUBJECTS AND ETHICAL ISSUES

Ethical conduct in research utilizing human subjects requires consideration of that individual's autonomy, right to privacy, and confidentiality. Federal government regulations require that institutional review boards (IRB) exist in universities and most medical care facilities that conduct research if these institutions receive federal funds. The IRBs are in place to balance the risks and benefits of research involving human subjects. Increasing human knowledge is not sufficient justification when risks are involved (Coughlin, 1997). Minimum standards include protecting the confidentiality or anonymity of patients, limiting access to raw data, protecting the patient's privacy, and utilizing the same level of confidence in conducting medical research as in the practice of health care (Edge and Groves, 1994). Certainly, results of such research should only be reported in an aggregate format; i.e., no identifiers should be reported.

Collection of personal information usually requires informed consent, so planning in advance is critical. However, not all research must be reviewed by these IRBs; e.g., quality assurance committees who are evaluating the quality and outcomes of care are usually exempt. Surveys and interviews of children are seldom exempt, and when students from outside the institutions are involved, IRB clearance is usually required. To be on the safe side, the local IRB with jurisdictions should be consulted.

Outcomes research needs data from patients/clients/customers. If we are following up on patients after treatment, we probably have access to name, addresses, and phone numbers. Before contacting them, we need to address the issue of confidentiality. Did the patients consent to being followed in a study? If our outcomes study is operating under the auspices of a quality improvement of the hospital, its medical staff, the medical group, or the health plan, we may not need explicit prior consent. Following up to determine patient outcomes after any treatment is an important part of any

[2]Lists of physicians are often obtained from medical societies who usually maintain lists of both members and non-members. There are several vendors who license the use of the American Medical Association Physician Masterfile and license researchers to use this data. Samples can be drawn based on physician demographics such as year of graduation and specialty as well as practice characteristics such as group, partnership, or solo practice. Other vendors have lists of other health-care professionals, hospitals, nursing homes, and other health-care organizations.

quality improvement function. However, if our survey research involves researchers who are not part of the quality improvement (QI) staff or who are from another institution, contact with the institutional review board, patient ethics, or human subjects committee of that organization is an essential first step.

SAMPLE SIZE CONSIDERATIONS

While planning, one of the first questions to ask is, "How big a sample size do I need?" As consultant, our usual response is, "That depends." While a complete discussion of sample size issues is beyond the scope of this chapter, we touch on several important considerations. Survey texts such as that of Aday (1996) provide excellent discussions along with straightforward methods to estimate the needed sample size. If you are not sure on this issue, you may want a statistical consultation before the survey. The number of completed surveys that would be needed to give the statistical power $(1 - \beta)$ and confidence (α) that we would ideally desire can be calculated using sample size formulas found in statistics books. In both descriptive and comparative situations, the smaller the measurement error or the smaller the difference between groups that you want to detect statistically, the greater the sample size needs to be. In our experience, we have seldom been able to afford the calculated sample size that the formulas suggest.

Like so many other things in survey research, identifying the sample size usually involves some type of compromise between statistical rigor and the realities of your budget. At the expense of being redundant, if you are not sure about this issue, seek out statistical consultation. An investment in this area before the survey will pay off. If fact, there are some situations when a statistical consultant may tell you that the large expensive sample you need is not really necessary to answer your research question in a defensible manner.

QUESTIONNAIRE DESIGN: COLLECTING RELIABLE AND VALID INFORMATION

The primary goal in designing a questionnaire is to allow respondents to provide reliable and valid answers to questions. *Reliable* means that information obtained is, within some definable limits of variation, the same answer every time you ask the question. Important types of reliability include day-to-day reliability, and reliability between multiple interviewers. A reliable questionnaire should get the same information from a respondent from day to day. Likewise, two interviewers should obtain the same responses from an interviewee. Sometimes the response to a single question or item on a questionnaire will not yield a reliable response, especially for questions of opinions or attitudes. To improve the reliability, multiple items that ask similar questions that "get at" the concept or attitude are included in the questionnaire. These multiple items are then added together or averaged to create a scale. Thus, it is common to create scales for attitudes, satisfaction, mental function mobility, etc. Statistical methods to determine the reliability of a scale exist with the Chronbach's alpha coefficient often used in publications to document a scale's reliability (Norusis, 1993).

To be a valid question, or series of them, questions must measure what they purport to measure. The truth or factual questions can be validated by checking source documents, such as medical records, or collecting the information from a second independent source that is known to be valid. The concept of validation is identical to the laboratory practice of comparing a new method to the "standard" method or "gold standard." Of course, if there is no agreement on a gold standard, you have to be more creative. For example, a patient's physical activity score can be validated by actually watching that patient do a specified task. Health status scores can be validated using physical examinations, laboratory tests, or a combination of performance tests and clinical opinions. Some measures may seek to predict future health status or risk. The predictive validity of an individual's poor self-rated health status could be validated by following clinic utilization, hospital admissions, or other outcomes over time. Attitudes and opinions are more difficult to validate. One way to validate a positive satisfaction rating regarding a service or product would be to determine if that patient, who had other options for obtaining the products or services, uses again in the future that product or service to which he or she gave a high rating. Validating is often a difficult and long-term endeavor. Again, whenever possible the best approach is to build your questionnaire with questions and scales that have been previously shown to be reliable and valid.

WHAT QUESTIONS TO ASK AND HOW TO ASK THEM

Facts versus opinions and attitudes. Assuming you are asking the right person, collecting factual information is more straightforward than collecting opinions, attitudes, and beliefs (Babbie, 1973). If collecting *facts* is the "science" of survey research, collecting *attitudes* is the "art." We commonly ask patients or physicians if they are "satisfied' with the services they have received. On the surface, satisfaction seems simple; however, it is a complex issue (Ahrony and Strasser, 1993). Take the example of a physician's level of satisfaction with laboratory services. The overall rating of satisfaction may be made up of a number of components, each related to a set of expectations. A physician may be perfectly satisfied with the laboratory's accuracy, having had no bad experiences that would lead him or her to believe that the analyses are anything but what they should be. On the other hand, several delays in reporting may have failed to meet the doctor's expectations and as a result the current opinion of the laboratory's turnaround time may be very low. When the same doctor is asked for "overall" satisfaction, how will the doctor respond? Some middle value? Or will the dissatisfaction with turnaround time or more recent experience pull the overall score? As can be seen here, general questions may often be answered based on a specific concern. Another concern with general questions is that they may not provide enough information so that the survey results can be used to help formulate a remedy for the "problem."

Patient outcomes are equally complex. A good example of a difficult outcome to measure precisely and accurately is pain. Extreme pain to one patient may be mild pain to another. Following an intervention such as surgery to replace a hip, how can we measure pain? Using an established general-purpose health status instrument such as the SF-36 (Ware, 1992) is useful, but it may not yield useful information if your study is attempting to measure relatively minor reductions in pain. Some researchers recognize this problem and have moved away from issues such as pain or feelings, preferring to measure functions that can be quantified. A common approach may be to ask how many days pain has kept them from completing their activities of daily living. In these situations, the best advice is to review the literature and use scales or questions that have been shown to be reliable and valid. Again, knowing the ultimate objective of the survey data will serve you well as you make decisions on how to measure outcomes.

OPEN- VERSUS CLOSED-ENDED QUESTIONS

There are some pros and cons to consider when selecting either the open-ended or closed-ended question format. The cons: Closed-ended questions tend to limit choices for the respondent. Or the choices that exist are not appropriate for the respondent—thus, always include an "other" category. Sometimes closed-ended questions would be too long or complicated to get at the possible answers; i.e., there are too many choices that would need to be present. Open-ended questions are difficult to code and subsequently analyze. Most frequently, open-ended questions are put into categories: categories that are created by the researcher, which may lead to serious bias. A questionnaire that incorporates only or a majority of open-ended questions will appear lengthy and burdensome to the respondent. This can dramatically affect response rates.

The pros: Closed-ended questions are relatively easy to code and utilize in subsequent analysis. They appear to the respondent to be easier and quicker to use. Open-ended questions are good when you want to allow the respondents to vent or you want to "catch" their opinions. They are also appropriate for those situations when little is known about the topic and you are collecting data that help establish a baseline of information.

PHONE OR MAIL SURVEY

One of the first decisions in planning the survey is the choice of a method(s) for distribution. In most situations, self-report mailed or telephone surveys are the common options. Qualitative interviews or less structured (open-ended) surveys also have an important place, primarily in exploring new areas or problems and preparing for larger scale quantitative surveys. In-person and group interviews, often called "focus groups," are essential to developing and pretesting questionnaires (Aday, 1996). Occasionally, quali-tative methods may be useful in exploring the "why" behind the numbers obtained on a survey. For smaller scale projects, face-to-face interviews may be considered, but for larger scale studies these are too expensive to be practical. Sometimes the budget or the situation (e.g., phone numbers but no addresses or vice versa) dictates the choice of method. Often investigators may need to explicitly consider the pros and cons of the phone versus mailed alternatives. Every survey research text that we know of lists criteria for selecting phone versus mail administration of questionnaires and discusses important pros and cons of each (Aday, 1996; Babbie, 1973). These should be consulted for more detail. Our experience is that a short list of relevant questions will point to the best method. These decision criteria should be applied as needed for a particular set of circumstances. The decision matrix in Table 1 lists some of the issues and situations that a project might confront and a brief rationale for a "best choice."

QUESTIONNAIRE FORMATTING: THE USER-FRIENDLY MAILED QUESTIONNAIRE

Formatting a mailed questionnaire. In concept it's simple: Make your question attractive (so it will be picked up and started), easy to read (so it is understandable and your respondent will continue), and easy to fill out (so that it is answered correctly). Many texts offer lists of suggestions, most of them good (Aday, 1996, Table 12.1). Again, focus on making it easy for the addressee to respond. Many research organizations have followed the trend toward questionnaires that are machine scannable, but this trend misses the essential point, which is to keep the questionnaire easy for the respondent. All things being equal, a tedious form tells the addressee, "Your time isn't as important as my lowering my data entry expenses." Think about your own experience: Scannable documents are tedious. This response format works best for a room of students who are taking a test. Ask your grandparent or a member of the medical staff if they will fill out a tedious questionnaire. Again, focus on the prime objective: Make it easy for the respondent. Spend a few more dollars to have the data key-entered from the questionnaire. The result will be a higher response rate and more valid information (Table 2).

INTERVIEWER-ADMINISTERED TELEPHONE QUESTIONNAIRES.

The critical issues for a telephone questionnaire (the script) are related to making the questions go smoothly and quickly. Computer-aided inter-

Table 1   Critical Issues in Choosing Between a Mailed Versus Phone Survey

Issue	Situation	Best choice
Is it possible to get the individual on the phone?	1. Physician has two offices and sees patients all day. You don't know of a block of time when she is at her desk.	Mail: It is almost impossible to administer phone surveys to physicians, but mailed surveys have lower response rates. Repeat mailings are essential.
	2. Patient is home during evening or on weekends—and your project has a good budget.	Phone: With repeated calls you can usually catch someone at home. Phone surveys usually have higher response rates than mailed surveys.
How complex is your questionnaire?	You have a branching questionnaire with different questions for patients mild versus severe disease.	Phone: It is the only choice when you have branching questions or subjects that will need help in understanding the question .
You have a limited budget.	1. You have time to do 2 or 3 mailings to get a higher response rate.	Mail: Surveys are usually much more economical; however, repeat mailings are needed for better response rate.
	2. You need the information soon.	No survey: It is better not to collect data if you can't do it in a manner that will yield valid results. Bad data are worse than no data. Some qualitative information from focus groups might help.
	3. You need the data next year.	Delay survey: Try to obtain resources to do a credible survey.
You are gathering facts, not attitudes or opinions.	You need facts on number of visits to the doctor, diet, medical expenses.	Mail or record review: If the respondent (individual or organization) must look up data, mail is usually better. Also consider gathering data from medical records.

Table 1 Critical Issues in Choosing Between a Mailed Versus Phone Survey *(continued)*

Issue	Situation	Best choice
You are gathering sensitive information.		Mail: Sensitive data or potentially negative opinions are best collected by mail. Calls from the hospital or health plan often obtain overly positive ratings because of our social norm to not say bad things. This is often called the "halo effect." Handing out satisfaction surveys at the clinic almost guarantees to yield very positive biased ratings. Consider an anonymous survey.

viewing (CAI) software that allows efficient branching during complex questionnaires is becoming more popular. Many large survey and market research firms use this technology. CAI systems also combine data entry with questionnaire administration so that turnaround times for getting reports can be almost instantaneous. Complete instructions for interviewers are especially essential for phone surveys. Employing multiple phone interviewers results in potential problems in standardization of responses. Having a script with standardized explanations, prompts, and probes is essential. Complete training and supervision are particularly critical during the early phases of interviewing. If possible, take more time to collect your data and use fewer interviewers to reduce this variation. Skilled interviewers are a critical variable to evaluate for when purchasing services from a vendor. For complex surveys, especially in multiple languages, avoid firms that depend on part-time employees who work on a per survey (piece) salary scale. If the survey is not complex, staff can perform the survey, and occasionally for some surveys volunteers can be effective. The key is good planning, from training to constant supervision during the administration of the phone survey.

CRITICAL SUCCESS FACTORS FOR ACHIEVING THE GOAL OF VALID INFORMATION

Avoiding the rush to collect data: Pretesting is the key. Pretesting is a critical step that must take place in a thoughtful and deliberate manner prior to sending or administering the questionnaire. Too often surveys go from the

Table 2   Some Key Ideas for Formatting Questionnaires

Issue	Notes and Comment
Grab attention with a concise cover letter.	Be sure to explain any tracking codes and assure respondents of confidentiality.
Provide clear instructions.	This is especially true when a respondent is asked to skip to or go to another question.
Consider the appearance carefully.	Use off-white colors; sometimes graphics may improve the appearance but don't be too cutesy.
Phrase full and complete questions.	Don't ask two questions at the same time. This is sometimes known as a "double-barreled" question.
Order questions to flow smoothly.	Keep similar questions together; build from basic to in-depth questions.
Minimize the number of pages.	But keep the font size large enough to read—11 or 12 points. The shorter the better, and the usual rule is no more than 4 pages.
Use closed-ended questions.	But always leave plenty of space to write "other" responses. The responses categories are often numbered (this is known as self-coding). Avoid this numbering if it makes the questionnaire appear too busy or cluttered.
Use open-ended questions, if needed.	Written comments provide a wealth of ideas and anecdotes, but categorizing and coding (known as postcoding) is labor-intensive and often unreliable.
End with a thank you.	Also be sure to include a self-addressed stamped envelope. Consider giving respondents a choice. Some respondents, especially organizations and physician offices, prefer to fax instead of mail back. This works well only for short questionnaires. Electronic mail response or a web-based response can be considered for some highly selected groups.
Deliver on promised incentives.	Too often we take too long to provide a summary report to respondents.

draft stage to administration in the "field" without adequate testing. The problem is often that even if the questions are clear to the investigators, the target audience may not understand them in the same way. Every discipline has its jargon, which should be avoided. If patients rather than professionals are being surveyed, there needs to be concern about the reading level. It is often recommended that general patient surveys be at about the eighth grade reading level. In some older or bicultural populations, the recommended levels may need to be even lower. If the questionnaire needs to be translated, the complexity of the research project is multiplied (Aday, 1996). Again, if this is required by the situation, allow extra time and significantly more resources.

The first rule is, always pretest in the target population, as opposed to graduate students or surgical residents in the lunch room. Pretest numbers do not need to be large; 10 to 20 are usually enough to detect problems and point toward improvements needed. The key is to do pretests systematically. Get the pretest individual to commit to completing the questionnaire as well as doing a verbal or written debriefing. In some cases you may want to conduct interviews prior to drafting questionnaire items. In-person and group interviews, sometimes-called "focus groups," are useful in developing and pretesting questionnaires, especially when the survey is new. It is useful to start with open-ended questions. Ask the question and wait for a response. This will also help determine what the common responses are likely to be, so that the finalized question potentially can include items to check off.[3]

Critical factor: Maximization of response rates. Always develop a protocol that will allow for follow-up mailings or phone calls. As noted earlier, three mailed (redundant) surveys are usually needed to attain the best possible response rate. For mailed surveys, our experience shows that only about 40% of those who ultimately responded did so on the first mailing (Hofherr et al., 1993). Persistence does pay off, and is one of the most critical variables in improving response rates. A minimum of five phone calls made at times when you expect the target group to be available is needed. It will come as no surprise that this usually means making calls between 5 and 8 p.m., around dinnertime for many families. Response rates have declined in recent years, perhaps due to the deluge of calls from the telemarketers wanting to give you yet another credit card. Answering machines and caller identification also make telephone calls more difficult. Calls during weekends and during the day may also be needed. As a practical matter, it is important to include identifiers on any mailed survey. This can be a number in a corner of the survey. The identifier is used to track responses so that those returning the survey are not sent surveys in follow-up mailings. Color coding the number allows you to determine which mailing they responded to. An explanation of this identifier should be given and the recipient should be assured it will only be used for tracking of responses for mailing and not linked with the survey contents.

Why is response rate important to the validity of survey results? Since the primary motivation for survey response is the interest in the topic, those who respond are likely to be the most highly motivated. For example, in a hospital satisfactions survey, the majority of early responders may be those at the extremes of dissatisfaction or satisfaction (John, 1992). As a rule,

---

[3]Copies of survey instruments and critique sheets for pretesting are available from the authors.

expect the first 20% to be highly biased one way or another. To generalize to the entire sampled group (the population) you need a much higher response rate. As described earlier, it is essential to compare respondents to the sampled population.

Critical factor: Incentives and response rates. Those who respond to surveys are different from those who don't. First and foremost, they are interested enough to take the time to complete the survey. If you want to increase the response rate, you need to gain the attention and keep the interest of the potential respondent. Incentives and persistence do work (Martin et al., 1989). For professionals, consider, at a minimum, sending the respondents a summary report from the survey. For patients and the general population, consider paying each respondent. Are there pens, flashlights, refrigerator magnets, discount coupons, or other token incentives that the project can afford? Will these incentives help to significantly increase the response rate? Build in the cost of the incentives when budgeting for the survey. Increasing interest and response is essential to the validity of your survey; spend time thinking of ways to improve the rate. Don't think of the cost of incentives as "add-ons" but in the context of the expenses for the entire survey. A 5–10% increase in expenses because of incentives or other methods to increase responses may yield a significant enhancement in the response rate and subsequently the validity of the survey.

ANALYSIS AND REPORTING INFORMATION: ISN'T THIS WHY WE ARE DOING THIS ANYWAY?

Data entry. Use software that you are comfortable with. The common database management packages for the PC work fine. Most are easy to learn, and files can be converted so that data can be imported into your statistical package. A public domain product, EPI-INFO, also has an easy-to-use data entry module (CDC Web Site, 1999). Quality control of your data should begin in the entry process. Databases allow you to set values that are valid for each variable entered. If your survey has open-ended responses, assure that this coding, which is often called postcoding, is done reliably. This may mean that two people need to code each survey and then check to assure that their categorizations agree.

Data preparation and analysis. Preparing data for analysis always takes more effort than you expect. Allow time and resources for the quality control of survey data. Carefully code variables that are skipped by some respondents. Don't code "skips" the same way you code "missing" variables that the respondent refused to complete or just left blank. Perform quality control checks to identify data entry errors that may have occurred. Values that are out of range or not logical can thus be identified and corrections can be made before final data analysis. Do this by reviewing an initial frequency distribution for all variables; this will help assure that you don't have unexpected codes. Cross-tabulations can aid in detecting illogical responses that may be coding or data errors. For any survey, don't neglect exploratory statistical analysis. Look at the distribution of all variables; don't assume that variables have normal distributions. These variables may need to be recoded into categories. PC-based statistical packages such as SPSS (Babbie, 1973) or SAS (SAS Institute, 1996) are easy to use and allow you to graphically examine all variables using a frequency histogram. Scatter plots between variables are also useful to examine relationships. Once the initial descriptive statistics are quality controlled, we have found it useful to fill in these data on a copy of the survey instrument. This serves as a useful reference to overall results of the survey for planning further bivariate analysis. As a guide to further statistical analysis, many statistical and survey research texts (Aday, 1996) provide excellent resources to assist in planning and executing tests of hypotheses.

CONCLUDING IDEAS

Collecting information from patients, professionals, and organizations is expensive and demanding work. Information gathered using surveys is increasingly important in order to make informed decisions for patients and our organizations. However, no matter what the problems and expenses, systematically collected valid data are essential to furthering institutional quality improvement goals, as well as disciplinary knowledge. In today's competitive marketplace, surveys are, for better or worse, an essential component in the way that health-care services will be rated and our organizations' performance graded.

The quality of surveys done in our work places and published in the literature varies greatly. As you read the results of a published survey or performance scorecard for consumers on the Internet, keep an open mind but reflect on some of the many factors that can compromise the reliability and validity of the information being presented. The topics discussed in this chapter should be helpful in identifying areas in which there may be concerns in the design, completion, and analysis of a survey, as well as potential biases. These critical factors should also be helpful when you hire someone to collect information that is needed to complete an outcomes research project.

RESOURCE APPENDIX: HELP FOR DOING SURVEY RESEARCH

Finding Help: Selecting a Consultant or Vendor

Consultants.   Market research and opinion polling organizations that perform surveys as their primary business can be quite helpful. Many of these firms are set up to do large surveys in a short period of time. The interviewers are usually not technically trained, so they don't introduce bias in the interview; the downside is that they can't answer questions for clarification. One-time research surveys require considerable "up-front" work and training of interviewers, and as a result purchasing services from this type of vendor can be very expensive.

Quick-and-dirty consultation.   Before hiring a consultant, take advantage of resources in your organization. Try different departments in your hospital or health plan. This might include a marketing department, a research department in a larger teaching hospital, or statisticians in an affiliated medical school. Most universities have faculty doing some type of survey research: psychology, marketing departments in a business school, public relations, sociology, etc. Many universities have survey research centers where expertise is available to help faculty and students who are doing surveys.

Selecting a consultant.   Purchasing survey services is not unlike buying any other service. The best predictor of a successful client–vendor relationship is good communication. If you know what you want, write it down. and communicate that to potential vendors, they should be able to respond with a meaningful proposal. Market research firms are widely available and often listed in the Yellow Pages. Other units in your organization may be able to refer you to a consultant. While some firms are "turn-key" operations that do everything, others may specialize in certain areas, such as collecting data, developing the survey instrument, or performing the analysis. What "package" of services do you want? Knowing what your survey is designed to collect is a good place to start, but how much assistance from a vendor or consultant will you need before and after the survey? Will you research the literature to find existing questionnaires that have been tested? Will you need more than one vendor? Using more than one vendor may, at times, be advantageous when each can contribute a different perspective; however, it may also be more work in negotiating and managing. Ultimately, you are the investigator and will need to take responsibility for the integrity of the survey and how the results are used, so even "turn-key" solutions cannot do everything.

Continuing to Learn More About Survey Research

Learn as much as you can from others by always starting with the published literature. Don't reinvent the survey. Build on the experience, success, and failure of others. If you can find an investigator who has worked in the field, most are willing to share their experience and instruments. Unfortunately, in the area of laboratory performance and outcomes measurement you will find little literature, but reports are being added. The Internet is filled with junk but there may be jewels, especially if you are considering an online survey. For any kind of patient survey involving health status, health-related quality of life, or other disease-specific outcomes, there are instruments aplenty (McDowell and Newell, 1996). Many specialized patient outcome surveys will be easy to find in the published literature. Surveys from CDC's National Center for Health Statistics also provide a large stock of questions for consideration for any health survey.

Increasing your survey savvy.   Reviewing a market research book is a good place to start (Kotler and Clarke, 1987). For a more in-depth look at health surveys, Aday's book (1996) is very complete and has everything most would want to know. There may even be Internet courses or course modules available online from college professors. Marketing departments may offer short courses and marketing professors may also serve as a potential source of expertise. The marriage of a laboratory researchers' content expertise with the general survey research knowledge of a graduate student or professor may be a good match.

REFERENCES

Aday L. *Designing and Conducting Health Surveys*, second edition. Jossey-Bass, San Francisco, 1996.

Ahrony L, Strasser S. Patient satisfaction: What we know about and what we still need to explore. *Med. Care Rev.* 1993;50:50–79.

Babbie ER. *Survey Research Methods*. Wadsworth, Belmont, CA, 1973.

Backstrom CH, Hursh GD. *Survey Research*. Northwestern University Press, Evanston, IL, 1963.

Centers for Disease Control, Epidemiology Program Office. Epi-Info Home page. June 1999 URL=http://www.cdc.gov/epo/epi/epiinfo.htm

Coughlin SS. *Ethics in Epidemiology and Public Health Practice. Collected Works.* Quill Publication, Washington, DC, 1997.

Edge RS, Groves JR. *The Ethics of Health Care. A Guide for Clinical Practice.* Del Mar Publisher, Cambridge, MA, 1994.

Hofherr LK, Peddecord KM, Benenson AS, Garfein RS, Francis DP, Cross JL, Rau J, Hewitt DJ. Physician experience with human immunodeficiency virus type 1 or hepatitis b testing in San Diego County: Methods for a census survey. *Clin. Lab. Sci.* 1993;6:110–115.

John J. Getting patients to answer: What affects response rates? *J. Health Care Market.* 1992;12:46–51.

Kotler P, Clarke R. *Marketing for Health Care.* Prentice-Hall, Englewood Cliffs, NJ, 1987.

Martin WS, Duncan WJ, Powers TL, Sawyer JC. Costs and benefits of selected response inducement techniques in mail survey research. *J. Business Res.* 1989;19:67–79.

McDowell I, Newell C. *Measuring Health: A Guide to Rating Scales and Questionnaires*, second edition. Oxford University Press, New York, 1996.

McLaughlin CP, Kaluzny A. *Continuous Quality Improvement in Health Care.* Aspen, Gaithersburg, MD 1994.

Norusis, MJ, SPSS, Inc. *SPSS Professional Statistics Users Guide*, Release 6.0. SPSS, Inc., Chicago, 1993.

Peddecord KM, Hofherr LK, Benenson AS, Garfein RS, Francis DP, Cross JL, Rau J. Use of a physician survey to identify opportunities for quality improvement. *Clin. Lab. Sci.* 1993;6:110–115.

Peddecord KM, Baron EJ, Francis DP, Drew JA. Quality perceptions of microbiology services: A survey of infectious diseases specialists. *Am. J. Clin. Pathol.* 1996;105:58–64.

Rau J, Cross JL, Hofherr LK, Peddecord KM, Benenson AS, Garfein RS, Francis DP. Physician satisfaction with HIV-1 and HBV testing in San Diego County. *Med. Care* 1996;34(1):1–10.

SAS Institute, Inc. *Getting Started With the SAS System Using SAS/ASSIST Software: Version 6*, 2nd edition. SAS Institute, Inc., Cary, NC, 1996

Ware JE. The MOS 36-item short-form health survey (SF-36): Conceptual framework and item selection. *Med. Care* 1992;30:473–483.

Chapter 6

The Construction and Usage
of Clinical Databases

R. D. Aller

WHAT OUTCOMES MEASURES ARE AVAILABLE?

The first issue to be addressed when one contemplates the construction of a clinical database is what outcomes measures exist that could be incorporated into the database. Of course, one should also incorporate structure and process indicators, so that one can establish correlations between certain processes and positive outcomes. However, we must attempt to measure the outcomes of the health-care system—and as laboratorians, we are well advised to identify, and measure, outcomes that arise in some way from our activities as pathologists and laboratorians.

One domain of activity in your organization is a natural source for outcomes measures and milestones: The clinical guidelines and pathways activity must show its validity and value through a positive impact on clinical quality measures and well-defined patient care milestones.

What types of outcomes measures are in use? At the risk of some redundancy with other chapters in this text, we provide some brief examples here. The outcome tracked for the longest time in public health and medicine is mortality; however, it is (fortunately) so infrequent that it rarely provides a useful quality improvement tool. To quote Ralph Korpman, "Human protoplasm is so rugged that you can give everyone on a ward a dose of digoxin they don't need—and only rarely will it actually kill a patient." Therefore, we must use measures of morbidity (illness)—or, conversely, try to quantitate health. A convenient mnemonic is the "five D's": death, disease, discomfort, dollars, and dissatisfaction.

Of particular importance in today's dollar-driven health-care system are measures to ensure that the managed care nonpayment system (a more apt term than a "payment" system!) is not harming patients. Examples include QualMed, in Pennsylvania, where if a screener turns down a procedure or medication, then there is a telephone follow-up, and a defined cascade of cross-checks to determine if that denial led to any adverse circumstances. In an increasing number of states, managed care companies can be held legally accountable for decisions that have a demonstrably adverse effect on outcome. In Missouri and other states, guidance of an HMO as the medical director is recognized as the practice of medicine (requiring a license to practice in the state). We hope that the public will demand measurable, accountable assurances that HMOs' financial shortcuts are not yielding adverse outcomes.

In certain circumstances, outcomes can even be used to make therapeutic decisions. Therapeutic trials are, in effect, on-the-fly outcomes studies. Off-the-cuff therapeutic trials are a particularly common (and useful) practice in pediatrics and in veterinary medicine (both instances where patient history and reports of symptomatology are difficult to elicit).

Classes of Outcomes

As physicians and laboratory scientists, we traditionally think of a single class of outcome—the physical/medical outcome. A binary death versus life is easy to measure, but (as noted earlier) not very useful. Morbidity—the occurrence of other undesirable diagnoses, such as infections and other complications—is our most common and also inadequate measure. Fortunately, our colleagues are now evaluating functional status, such as the New York Heart cardiac classification, or the ability to ambulate a year after hip replacement surgery. Going a step further, a variety of measures of "quality-of-life" are now being used.

A second class of outcome, much more challenging to quantitate, is the psychological outcome: How does the patient and family feel about their health? Many commonly performed laboratory studies impact more on psychology—by risk factor assessment, knowing your prognosis—than on traditional "medical" outcome.

A third class of outcome is satisfaction. This is a consideration not only for the patient—but also for their family. As providers of service to many professionals within the health-care system, laboratorians need to be also measuring physician, nursing, administration, and even third-party payor satisfaction.

In evaluating patient satisfaction, we should remember that the major sources of patient dissatisfaction in most health-care organizations are not medical or technical; they are fundamental issues of ease of access, bedside manner and courtesy, hotel service, and waiting time. How much attention do we devote in our own organizations to addressing these areas?

A crude, after-the-fact surrogate measure of dissatisfaction with some prepaid health plans is the rate at which patients and their families switch *out* of the health plan at the next reenrollment period.

Those who think that the satisfaction dimension can be given short shrift, in favor of the "best medical quality," should remember that a dissatisfied patient is far more likely to bring a malpractice action. The best medical quality in the world is no protection: Some remarkable recent research reveals that the amount of malpractice dollar awards correlates with disability result, not with actual malpractice (as judged by an independent panel of experts, reviewing a series of charts).

A fourth and final class of outcome is financial. These outcomes are extensively measured—indeed, every one of our organizations is driven by a certain type of financial outcome (net revenue vs. cost), often to the neglect of measuring medical and satisfaction outcomes. The dollars directly spent by the third-party payor, or the employer, are usually very carefully measured. Unfortunately, other financial impacts—which may be much larger—are often ignored. What is the impact of the patient's illness, in terms of lost work hours? What is the cost on a population-wide basis? What is the cost to society? What is the effect of this expenditure over a 20-year time frame (instead of the 3- to 5-year horizon favored by most accountants). This lack of perspective results in outrageous discrepancies such as huge Medicare expenditures in the last year of life, while childhood immunization programs are unfunded.

Types of Outcomes

Outcomes also vary in how directly and immediately they can be linked to a causative factor. Proximate outcomes are clearly the result of a particular intervention (or misadventure). Intermediate outcomes, such as hospital length of stay, or cost of an admission, are more commonly measured. Final outcomes measure patient function at the (expected) conclusion of an episode of illness. As before, the "ultimate" outcome—death—is measurable, but not often useful in most quality improvement efforts. As one moves down this scale, one quickly reaches the point at which it is difficult to determine if this outcome is at all attributable to your intervention.

Value of an Outcome

Value is typically described as the quotient of quality, divided by cost. Indeed, many interventions are evaluated in the research literature in terms of "cost per quality-adjusted year of life saved." Such measurements depend heavily on "quality of life." Standard measures such as the SF-12 and SF-36 scales are commonly used. However, the only valid judges of "quality of life" are the patients themselves. Different people have very different values systems, and what to one person is an overwhelming disability or devastation may to another be relatively minor. A glaring example of this disconnect is seen in the management of cancer patients on chemotherapy. Most oncologists think that their patients find cancer pain most disabling—yet most cancer patients find the cancer- and chemotherapy-associated fatigue far more troubling.

In considering quality of life, we would be well served to remember the comment by Yale's Paul Beeson, commenting on the palliative rice diet given patients in end-stage renal failure before the availability of renal dialysis—"Are we actually prolonging this person's life, or are we only making it seem longer?"

Prognostic Indicators

Many expensive new laboratory determinations are justified on the basis that they allow the clinician to better predict the outcome of the patient. How useful is this? Clearly, this is useful if it will enable the clinician to make a different (better) therapeutic or management decision than he or she would have been able to do without the indicator. Even if therapy or management remains unchanged, it may be useful to the patient in knowing what to expect for the future. They may allay anxiety—but how much of this is a placebo effect, just like the clinic in Mexico?

Unfortunately, many conditions have such a variable outcome, even given a certain level of a prognostic indicator, that they are of no value when counseling the patient. There is a great fallacy in attempting to use a useful epidemiological tool in the management or prediction of an individual patient.

WHAT MEASURES SHOULD WE USE?

Given that there are thousands of potentially useful measures, which shall we choose? The first choice, as we have just noted, is between statistically valid measures that enable us to say useful things about entire populations, and those that are useful in the individual patient's evaluation. As this is a text in medical outcomes, not on public health, we concentrate on the latter.

The most important criterion, in selecting outcomes measures for incorporation into a clinical database, is to find measures that can be gathered efficiently. What data can we readily acquire, without undue pain? This is colloquially referred to as "the low-hanging fruit." The liberally funded health-care institutions of the past are ancient history—we no longer have underutilized pathology residents, medical technology students, secretaries, or other "peons du jour" to do our "scut work." We must maximize the efficiency of ourselves and our staff as we gather these measures. To be useful, an outcomes database must be longitudinal—gathered over a prolonged time period. No matter how well intentioned you may be at their inception, labor-intensive measures will not be maintained long enough to be useful.

The other key aspect of selecting an outcome is to address a process about which something can be *done*. Is the system amenable to standardization, intervention, or reduction in variability? If you had not noted it elsewhere, it is worthwhile mentioning that, by itself, reduction in variability of a process usually equates to an increase in quality of outcome. Is a good therapy available for this disease? Is there a reliable way to prevent occurrence or progression of this disease process? In essence—can I take action? By measuring this outcome, can I close the loop?

WHERE DO WE OBTAIN THE DATA?

The most immediate and useful source of data for our clinical outcomes database is our own laboratory information system. However, one should not make the error of assuming that the data we want will be there when we need it. Laboratory information systems (LIS) are typically designed and optimized for the day-to-day function of the laboratory. Often, data that would be most helpful for outcomes studies are "purged" soon after the laboratory test has been performed, or within weeks of the patient's discharge from the hospital. As soon as feasible, one should begin downloading all patient, order, and result data from the LIS into one's own separate database, where it can be maintained permanently. Typically, this information can be extracted using LIS vendor-supplied tools, downloaded as a "flat file," then loaded into PC-based tools.

Hospital Data

A second source of useful information is the general hospital information system. Surprisingly, billing and other financial data can provide quite a bit of outcomes-related information, such as what procedures were necessary in a given patient (e.g., to deal with a complication). Regrettably, many hospitals and health systems have gone overboard in trying to use financial information for clinical purposes. For example, attempts are commonly made to correct for severity of illness by highly indirect measures, such as how much was spent to care for the patient.

One source of data to *avoid* in an outcomes database is the extraction of information from the paper medical record. This may seem counterintuitive, since so many of our studies in the past have relied on poring through vast mounds of paper, but there are two compelling reasons to avoid depending on the paper chart: The most important problem is the poor quality of data usually recorded in charts. The chart contains no mechanism to detect or prevent errors. While errors of commission might be noted by those reading the chart, the more serious problem of omitted data is far more difficult to detect. The second problem is the difficulty and cost (noted earlier) of gathering data that are not in machine-readable form.

One should then seek out other information systems, or sources of electronic information, within the health-care system. Information systems serving radiology, pharmacy, respiratory-care, dietary, the operating room, and many other departments will provide a wealth of information. Although you should seek it out and attempt to use it, beware of the data in the medical records abstracting subsystem. Since abstract data are typically derived after the fact from the paper chart, rather than generated prospectively as a by-product of the care process, they are likely to be less reliable than other clinical data. Certainly, if data are available from a electronic medical records system, or a clinical data repository, those should be incorporated into your repository.

Certain systems in the health-care enterprise are already focused on the collection and analysis of outcomes data. Do not overlook infection control, quality assurance/quality improvement studies and systems, and satisfaction survey systems. Severity systems based on clinical parameters, such as APACHE, are extremely useful; interestingly, the most predictive parameters in these environments are often laboratory values! Another outcome-related database that is long established and can, in the appropriate context, be a highly useful data source is the tumor registry.

The Continuum of Care

While it may be easiest to acquire data from within the hospital environment, the database must encompass the entire continuum of care of the patient to be very useful. Hospital data, out of the longitudinal context, do not tell you very much. For example, an isolated hemoglobin of 4 gm/dl may have widely different significance—in one case, a discharged cardiac surgery patient, who declined transfusions, is doing fine (albeit rather fatigued). Critical and actionable laboratory values vary by specialty—the primary care physician depends on us to call values that we would never dream of calling to the oncologist. This is yet another way in which the pathologist can add value for the primary care provider: by providing specialty consultation without inconvenience or capitation penalty.

Databases assembled by integrated health-care systems, such as the Kaiser-Permanente system, will be key to their ability to prevail in the competitive health-care environment. Kaiser has been investing many millions of dollars to optimize the structured nomenclature it will be using to gather and understand clinical data; it will have orders of magnitude better data on care process, and true quality of care, than its less integrated competitor "HMOs."

Third-Party Comparative Databases

Very useful assemblages of data are available from a variety of third parties, and from the central offices of mega-systems. Where feasible, extractions from these databases should be made, and loaded into the laboratory outcomes database system.

These data may simply be a reprocessing of data acquired from your institution's information sources, formatted for more effective analysis. Examples of such products include the offerings of Transition Systems, Inc., and McKesson HBOC's Trendstar tool. There are many other examples of "managed care" and "decision support" software, which commonly takes such an approach.

Data compiled from many facilities within a hospital system or organization are often available to compare performance between different institutions. Columbia/HCA maintains a large database of this type, and the University Healthcare Consortium makes available to its membership a useful comparative tool; in late 1996 this already required a 9-gigabyte local disk to load the summarized database content. Other systems provide comparison and benchmarking tools for their membership. Again, extracting aspects of this data for use in the laboratory clinical database is recommended.

Several companies assemble data from a variety of nonaligned hospitals, and sell this as a comparison and benchmarking tool. Some of these companies, such as HCIA, drive their data extraction off governmental and public data sources. Others, such as MediQual's Pennsylvania quality index, base their systems on more extensive data extraction by member hospitals.

Beware of the large benchmarking databases, however. In many cases, they rely primarily or exclusively on financial and billing data, not clinical findings. Many claim to measure outcomes, but the only outcomes they can reliably address are mortality, cost, and a few complications with very well-defined coding parameters. They do *not* have sufficient clinical data to guide changes in clinical process—which is our best mechanism to improve outcomes.

Government Published and Distributed Data

Don't overlook direct use of large governmental data sources. Some of the most important outcomes findings ever published in laboratory medicine were derived from such sources. For example, Winkelman studied Medicare billing tapes, and discovered that patients receiving prothrombin time testing in low-volume laboratories (e.g., physician's office labs) were twice as likely to *die* within two weeks of the test as those who had been tested in a high-volume laboratory. Of course, one must keep in mind the intrinsic limitations of data that have been gathered for billing and reimbursement purposes.

Again, we should look beyond hospital discharge data. For example, in Pennsylvania, mandated collection and government reporting of data includes HMOs, and licensed ambulatory health-care facilities such as surgicenters and emergicenters.

DATA LINKAGE

Once data have been gathered from a wide variety of electronic sources, a major challenge remains before they can be used to track a person's progression through an episode of illness, to an outcome—one must determine which data belong to which person. Within a well-centralized hospital, most data will be identified by a medical record number—unless it has been mistyped, or omitted. In the past, the medical record number usually included a check digit (a digit, usually at the end of a record number, which is itself calculated from the other digits in the number), which permitted validation and helped prevent transposition errors. Unfortunately, many hospitals have discontinued using check digits, having the delusion that online entry of data would eliminate the need for self-checking record numbers.

Unfortunately, the venue for our most critical studies, of longitudinal outcome within the community setting, does not have any such coherent medical record number. We must make do with a variety of unsatisfactory substitutes.

Our Canadian colleagues have the advantage of a province-wide health identifier number. While not universally used, and less helpful when patients move between provinces or receive part of their care in the United States, this is orders of magnitude better than the mess in the United States.

A number of proposals have been made over the years to use the U.S. Social Security number as a health-care linkage tool. Indeed, in certain settings, such as GYN cytology databases (patient name being intrinsically unreliable in this setting, with the tradition of women changing their name upon marriage or divorce), the Social Security number has been shown useful. However, it has many limitations, such as its nonuniqueness (perhaps several hundred thousand individuals have duplicative social security numbers), its absence for some indigent populations, and its absence for children. Others have presented a detailed support, and critique, of the Social Security number as a health-care identifier.

In 1996, Congress passed the Healthcare Insurance Portability and Accountability Act, which had many important provisions for medical information management. In addition to requiring standard formats for many electronic billing transactions, it mandated that a plan be developed for a universal patient identifier. Regrettably, subsequent Congressional action to move forward on the universal patient identifier engendered public hue and cry over confidentiality issues. Somehow, members of the public seems to think they will be better off if it remains impossible to assemble a coherent picture of an individual's health history, and are skeptical of privacy safeguards that have been so far proposed.

Even if Congress tomorrow mandated the establishment of a national health identification number, the sheer magnitude and complexity of the task would consume many billions of dollars, and would take close to a decade to implement. Therefore, for practical purposes, we must move forward without near-term prospect of a solution to the patient linkage problem.

How do you assemble the data, in the meantime? Find a colleague in your Health Information Department (what used to be called "medical records") who is expert in patient linkage. If such a person is unavailable, you may need to seek outside consulting support. In either case, obtain patient-master-index and linkage software to carry you forward. It may be most practical to contract with an outside service bureau to perform linkage on your existing several years of historical data, then bring in-house the expertise to keep this linkage up to snuff as data are added prospectively. Going forward, try to make sure as many systems as possible are, at the data entry front end, driven off an enterprise-wide master person index.

DATA QUALITY, VALIDITY, AND CONFIDENTIALITY

Garbage in, garbage out: so phrased was the realization, at the dawn of the computer age, that the most sophisticated analysis tools in the universe are useless if the raw data is flawed. Predictably, much of the data you acquire and load into the laboratory outcomes database will be faulty. Data are dirty until they are used. If no one is using the contents of a data field, the quality of data entry into that field will inevitably deteriorate. One recent example: A laboratory began using a download of all laboratory orders to begin tracking phlebotomist workload. The first reports revealed that the phlebotomy supervisor was drawing 80 patients per day, while several of the phlebotomists were only drawing one or two. When investigated, those keying in records from the morning draw and other phlebotomy rounds explained that if they couldn't read the initials of the phlebotomist on the labels/tube, they had been simply putting in the supervisor's number—no one had ever complained, so they figured this was fine! With their understanding that the data were now being *used*, data quality improved dramatically.

A second basic principle is that data are suited for the purpose motivating their collection. Therefore, billing data are aimed solely at preparing a bill. When such data are misapplied to tease out clinical information, or even to try to judge severity of illness, the results (although widespread) are often not much better than a random number generator.

The most troubling error in health-care data is the error of omission. Unless there is a tight link and close coupling between the existence of a finding and its recording into the electronic records system—and we are fortunate that we do have such a coupling in most laboratories—then the absence of a finding from the database may mean any one of several things: It wasn't looked for; it was looked for, but wasn't present, but the observer didn't think it important to document; it was looked for, and was present, but the observer didn't think it had anything to do with the disease process that the observer was looking at; or it was looked for, was present, and was documented—but in a format that is not intelligible to our database parser.

The Paper Medical Record as a Paradigm of Suboptimal Data

The paper medical record can be used as a prime example of almost everything to avoid in a data source. The fidelity of data transmission (legibility) is lacking. Indeed, some claim that premed students are given a handwriting exam before admission to medical school, and those with the most illegible handwriting admitted; I personally believe, though, it is intensified by the first portion of medical school, during which one attempts to write notes continuously for 8–10 hours a day, for 2 years.

A much larger problem is completeness—there is no mechanism to ensure that all pertinent information relating to a diagnostic or management situation is asked the patient, or recorded in the chart. Often, "shadow" charts exist containing the physician's direct impressions, and the "official" medical record encompasses only a collection of data of secondary importance.

Availability of and access to the medical record is another major hurdle. One of Korpmans' Laws of Medical Systems states: Wherever the patient is, the chart isn't! Why does the patient have to wait 4 hours to begin a 30-minute chemotherapy infusion? Because the chart, containing the only extant copy of the physician's orders, is stuck in the wall in a broken-down transport trolley! The shadow charts noted earlier exist primarily because the physician needs to be assured of immediate access to his or her experience with this patient—not to be dependent on taking the hours or days to find an overstuffed and largely irrelevant (for that subspecialty) sheaf of material.

Which portions of the paper record are particularly gaping holes? Regrettably, just those data types that exist *only* in the paper chart, such as patient history (particularly beyond the current chief complaint), physical exam (especially when it lies outside the primary specialty of the physician), and "secondary" diagnoses—which may be highly significant to the patient, but are not those being immediately managed at this moment. Most charts have complete and accurate versions of laboratory data, radiology reports, and the like—but most physicians don't *use* the charts for this latter data, finding that direct access to the computer is even more accurate, complete, and rapid.

Retrospective Versus Prospective Data

Most data that we accumulate into our clinical database will likely be retrospective, gathered before we knew exactly for what purpose it was being collected. Prospective data will take longer to gather (since it isn't already collected), but is likely to be of higher quality/usefulness, since it can be oriented and sufficiently detailed for the research question. The detailed design of data collection instruments is beyond the scope of this chapter, but a few general principles should be mentioned: Design the instrument first as a paper questionnaire—even though it should not be used in production in that form—and try it on a few cases to detect design errors. Don't attempt to collect data that are extraneous, or superfluous.

Indeed, a properly designed and configured electronic medical record system can serve as a general-purpose prospective data-gathering tool, focused on aspects that we know to be routinely deficient in the paper medical record. The mechanisms for provider interaction must be highly efficient, or the record system will not be used.

So We Have a Measurement—and We See a Change—Does That Mean Anything?

An isolated change in any outcomes measure—no matter how dramatic—has no significance unless you know the historical variability of that measure. One must gather a *number* of data points on any given "outcome measure," before one can distinguish between continuing random variation, and an effect of an intervention. One does well to remember Ernest Witebsky's comment, circa 1958, about a sample of one—"wun mouse is no mouse"

You *must* establish a baseline of performance before changing things. The most important measurement period during any outcome or quality improvement study may well be before you have made any system changes or introduced any interventions. Study random variability of the process over time. *Then* introduce an intervention. Is there a statistically significant change in the "outcome measure"? Even if the median—or mean—hasn't shifted significantly, one can rejoice in a significant decrease in the variability of that outcome measurement. In general, processes with a reduced variation are higher quality processes.

Do You Have Legal Access to the Data You Are Studying?

Until recently, most of us would have assumed that if we had physical access to a group of data, as part of our ordinary occupation, we could analyze that data and draw conclusions (of course, always omitting disclosure of any patient identities as the results are published). Remarkably, human studies committees and institutional review boards are now interpreting confidentiality regulations even more stringently. One group performing some very exciting work on laboratory data mining has been delayed in publishing the findings of their studies because data access permissions had not been clearly defined/elucidated before the studies were done.

We have a legal and moral obligation to the patients we serve, to safeguard the confidentiality of that data, wherever we might retain it—including in a laboratory outcomes database. Beyond our scope in this chapter, we refer the reader to the large (and rapidly growing) body of literature on this issue.

The HIPAA regulations, noted earlier, also will have far-reaching impact in requiring more stringent safeguards of patient data confidentiality. Some have suggested that this is the next "Y2K problem" to strike the world of medical information systems.

KEY CHARACTERISTICS OF THE OUTCOMES DATABASE

We have devoted most of this chapter to decisions about what goes into the outcomes database; now we consider how it should be built and maintained.

Standard Nomenclature/Reference Terminology

It is essential that as much as possible of the data loaded in should be acquired, and maintained, in a standard, structured format. Rather than gathering clinical observations and findings as mounds of free text, we strongly advocate that this be codified into a standard nomenclature or reference terminology. Until recently, there was some debate in medical informatics about the best tool for the job. The recently announced merger of SNOMED (Systematized Nomenclature of Medicine) and the READ code (used by the British National Health Service for tracking all ambulatory and acute care episodes) settles this debate. With the investment by Kaiser of several million dollars to improve the Reference Terminology capabilities of SNOMED, our path forward is evident. Wherever feasible, the nomenclature/reference terminology should be built in to the clinical front end of any system, so that clinical observations can be captured directly in the most specific, pertinent concepts. Postprocessing of freely dictated physicians' notes is extremely problematic.

Technical Considerations

Those who turned to this chapter looking for a treatise on relational database structures and the third-normal form have doubtless given up by now—but we do need to devote some attention to the technical underpinnings of these systems.

The logical choice for most situations would be to load your data into a standard relational database. These are commercially available from a variety of sources, and range from relatively light-duty tools such as Microsoft Access, to industrial-strength programs such as Oracle, Sybase, Microsoft SQL Server, Unify, Informix, and others. Your best bet would be to go with a database with which your organization already has experience, and for which there are staff members who can provide you with support and guidance. Your hospital may have a site license for Oracle, or may have standardized on another tool. There would rarely be circumstances where you would want to deviate from the institution-standard approach.

However, it is worthwhile noting that you should expect the database to reach multi-gigabyte size. Light-duty tools such as Access may not have the horsepower to handle this.

In the longer term, or if your institution has begun moving in this direction, use of an object-oriented database may confer significant advantages of efficiency and effectiveness. Again, seek the counsel of your local information systems support staff.

If your institution is running applications written in M, or using the next-generation relational and object tools of Cache, you may wish to consider hosting your database on this platform. M makes extremely efficient use of the hardware platform, and can serve as an effective outcomes database tool if a sufficient number of indexes are built, to the fields you are likely to search on. On the other hand, it will not offer as large a range of statistical and other tools to analyze the data.

The database should be configured so that it can be accessed from multiple workstations within the laboratory, rather than requiring anyone who wishes to make a query to use a single workstation. Therefore, the database folder must be shared across the local area network.

Wherever possible, the data should be stored in a structured, encoded form, rather than as free-text or free-form entries. Free text is extremely difficult to process, and free-form entries can assume such a wide variety of possible values that analysis and grouping of cases will be exceedingly difficult.

There are a variety of technical tools that may be used for analysis of the data, such as chi-square, cluster analysis, and the whole class of techniques grouped under the term "data mining." We do not attempt here to present a glossary of statistical and analysis techniques, but refer the reader to the next chapter, as well as to any of the excellent textbooks on analysis of large datasets.

Indeed, we would predict that you will find the principal impediments to usefulness of your clinical outcomes database to be incompleteness, imprecision, and invalidity of data, rather than lack of technical and analysis tools.

WHAT TO DO WITH THE FINDINGS FROM YOUR OUTCOMES DATABASE

When contemplating the construction of a laboratory clinical outcomes database, one must be clear on the objectives. Our view is that this database will enable the organization to maintain and improve patient care, while undertaking interventions that also enable cost reduction.

My basic philosophy is that we are here to serve the patient—the clinician helps us understand what the patient needs. There is no question that our health-care system will have fewer dollars tomorrow to care for patients than we had yesterday. Under these circumstances, there is only one approach that is clearly unacceptable: that is to do things the same way we have always done them. To improve patient outcome—or even to maintain it—we *must* change continually.

However, while change is clearly mandatory, improvement is optional. Overwhelming changes in the payment system and the organization of medical care will continue to occur. We *must* have metrics in place, and follow these metrics in a database we control, to ensure that the externally forced changes are not impairing patient outcome. Meaningful and constructive change has a net vector—it is not a random walk.

Beware of buzzwords. Patients become clients, and physicians become providers. The abysmal orientation of the insurance industry is made clear by their term "medical loss ratio" to refer to all expenditures that provide any benefit to the patient, in terms of patient care!

In addition to the crucial and central role described in this chapter for computerized databases of outcomes, information systems are probably of even more importance in the outcomes arena in being effector agents for the implementation of change. We pathologists must continue to reassert our role as the physician's physician. Leadership is the management of change for positive outcomes. Outcomes metrics are essential to know that the changes you are leading are actually improvements. Keep pursuing the goal!

Chapter 7

Data Mining and Knowledge Discovery

S. A. Moser and S. E. Brossette

BACKGROUND

Over the last quarter century, our ability to collect and store data has grown faster than our ability to analyze data. By current estimates, the world's data amount doubles every 20 months (Frawley et al., 1992). This data proliferation has created a demand for new, semiautomatic methods for extracting useful information from data to facilitate modeling, surveillance, scientific discovery, quality control, and decision making processes. Today, *data mining* answers this demand.

Data mining is the partially automated process of finding potentially interesting, previously unknown patterns in data. The goal of data mining is to uncover deposits of useful patterns in complex data that would otherwise require large amounts of time, resources, or luck using traditional hypothesis-driven methods. These findings can be used (1) to support mission-critical decision making, (2) for prediction and classification tasks, (3) for summarization, (4) for surveillance, or (5) to explain observed phenomena (McDonald et al., 1998). Data mining lives at the interface of database technology, machine learning, graphics, statistics, and a diverse set of application domains. Early in the development of the field, a distinction was made between *data mining* and *knowledge discovery* in databases (KDD). KDD represents the overall process, while data mining refers to a tool used in the process of knowledge discovery. Today, the two have become synonymous and the term *data mining* is usually used.

Data mining has certain advantages over traditional methods. In traditional knowledge discovery, one has a hunch, formulates a hypothesis, collects data, summarizes it, computes a test statistic, and interprets the statistic with respect to a known probability distribution. The hunch sometimes originates from a structured analysis of descriptive statistics. More often, however, it is constructed in an ad-hoc fashion based on intuition. For relatively small, low-dimensional data, this type of manual hypothesis-driven knowledge discovery works well, and well-worn statistical programs can handle the data efficiently. For modern databases, however, which frequently contain millions of records and gigabytes of high-dimensional data, traditional methods are futile. Consequently, subtle and complex patterns are never suspected and go undiscovered.

Extensive reviews of the data mining technique can be found in Fayyad et al. (1992, 1996) and John (1997). Statistical considerations in data mining are reviewed by Hand (1998).

THE DATA MINING PROCESS

Data mining is an iterative and interactive process centered on the interaction between a domain expert and an analyst. While the exact structure of the process differs from one description to another, it consists of the following basic steps (John, 1997) .

Understand the Problem

Although this seems obvious, it can't be overstated. The problem is usually well understood by the domain expert, but not by the analyst. Conversely, data mining is usually well understood by the analyst but not by the domain expert. Therefore, before a data mining project can be successfully deployed, a problem must be defined, a target data set must be identified, the desired types of mined patterns must be specified, and both the domain expert and the analyst must have an understanding of the desires and capabilities of the other.

Extract the Data

Target data sets usually reside in one or more transaction or operational databases. These databases are usually used for purposes other than analysis. Therefore, before they can be used for data mining, special data marts or data warehouses must first be created to contain selected data from disparate systems. Once these central analysis-centered databases are created, data can be extracted from them to feed to data-mining algorithms. Sometimes the data are so abundant that sampling schemes are employed to reduce the time and resource requirements necessary to analyze them. Sampling is discussed throughout the statistics literature, and is being looked at closely in some data mining problems.

Clean/Engineer the Data

Once the appropriate data have been identified and consolidated in easily accessible data marts and data warehouses, they need to be cleaned to remove bad data. This is usually accomplished via queries that perform sanity checks against the data in order to remove contaminated records. Other data engineering activities include attribute selection, to select only those attributes that are going to be useful, and variable transformation, to convert the values of a particular attribute into others that are more informative.

Select a Data-Mining Algorithm and Use It to Search for Patterns

Data-mining algorithms are of two basic varieties: predictive and descriptive. Predictive or classification algorithms construct models that predict the value of a given attribute based on the values of other attributes within the same data set. These algorithms include those that construct regression models, neural networks, decision trees, and classification rules. Regression models are used when the target (predicted) attribute is real-valued. Neural networks, decision trees, and classification rules can be used for both nominal and real-valued targets. All of these models can be verified by testing against data that was not used in their creation.

The second class of algorithm, the descriptive algorithm, generates patterns that are used to provide insight into problem domains. Association rule generators and clustering algorithms are most notable in this class.

Evaluate the Results

Pattern evaluation must be conducted by domain experts, and feedback must be given to the analyst so that revisions in previous steps can be made. This process of evaluation, feedback, and refinement is crucial for the success of a data mining project. The goal is to have a system that produces patterns that are manageable in number, and useful enough to justify the time required by domain experts to evaluate them. These problems are statistical in nature and require some statistical consideration. Briefly, data-mining algorithms search for unexpected, potentially interesting patterns and therefore perform many tests—one for each candidate pattern. These tests, called multiple comparisons, have been widely criticized by statisticians because they generate too many false positive results—patterns that are statistically significant, but really describe just normal chance fluctuations in the data. The resulting problem, too many patterns, is hardly better than the original problem, too much data.

While it is true that the careless application of data-mining algorithms often results in an overabundance of spurious and uninteresting findings—pattern glut—well-planned data mining projects successfully deal with pattern glut and yield a manageable set of results that can be reviewed in a timely and efficient manner. While some uninteresting patterns are inevitable in all data-mining projects, too many can make their evaluation cumbersome and unmanageable. For this reason, data mining requires careful planning, user interaction, evaluation, and refinement for its success.

APPLICATIONS

Data mining is being applied successfully in a number of different domains. For example, data are mined to determine sales and inventory patterns (Anand and Kahn, 1992), to detect fraudulent credit card activity (Blanchard, 1994), and to develop stock selection strategies (Hall et al., 1996; John, 1997). Additionally, satellite image data are mined for earthquake patterns (Shek et al., 1996), and even basketball statistics are mined to help identify important match-ups in upcoming games (IBM, 1995).

In health care and the biological sciences, there have been relatively few data-mining ventures. A Medline search spanning 1966 to the present using the terms "data mining" or "knowledge discovery" produced only 57 citations. Among these, Matheus, Piatetsky-Shapiro, and McNeill (1996) describe the KEFIR system, which identifies possible cost-saving measures based on deviations in preselected health outcomes, and several groups describe statistical and machine learning techniques that generate diagnostic and prognostic rules from clinical data sets (Prather et al., 1997; Tsai et al., 1997; Tsumoto et al., 1995). Basic science applications include mining molecular sequence data for structural motifs (Holfacker et al., 1996) and predicting a protein's secondary structure from its primary structure (Alnahi and Alshawi, 1993).

Only a few systems have been developed and applied to the laboratory medicine domain. The primary examples assist in infection control surveillance. These include the Computerized Infectious Disease Monitor (CIDM) based on the HELP system developed by LDS Hospital (Burke et al., 1991; Evans et al., 1986; Rocha et al., 1994), GermWatcher© developed at Barnes Hospital at Washington University (Kahn et al., 1993, 1996a, and 1996b), and the Data Mining Surveillance System (DMSS) developed at the University of Alabama at Birmingham (Brossette et al., 1998; Moser et al., 1999; Wong et al., 1997).

The CIDM system uses an integrated patient medical record (HELP) that contains laboratory, radiology, pharmacy, patient demographics, and clinical data to predict patients at risk for acquiring nosocomial infections. It does so daily by utilizing predetermined criteria established by domain experts and regression analysis. While the system identified 63% of patients with nosocomial infections (Evans et al., 1992), no evaluation of effect on patient outcomes was performed.

GermWatcher, unlike CIDM, is an expert system that relies on a restricted data set, the results of microbiology laboratory testing, to identify possible nosocomial infections. The system then undergoes rule adjustments based upon the ranking of the output by infection control nurses and an infectious disease physician. These adjustments improve system performance over time (Kahn et al., 1996a). The authors have found that the system increases the efficiency of infection control surveillance at Barnes Hospital, but like CIDM, a significant false positive rate negates some of the benefit.

Neither CIDM nor GermWatcher is in general use, although they have existed for 10 and 5 years, respectively. More importantly, both of these approaches require patterns of interest to be known before monitoring activities begin. Thus, patterns and relationships that are not known to be of interest in advance will go undetected.

DMSS AS A PROTOTYPICAL DATA MINING APPLICATION

Traditionally, hospital infection control surveillance includes a manual review of suspected cases of nosocomial infection followed by the tabulation of basic summary statistics. Antimicrobial resistance surveillance consists of the construction of periodic (i.e., annual or semiannual), hospital-wide antibiogram summaries that contain percent susceptibilities per organism/drug combination. Such summaries are not timely and often mask emerging, complex patterns (Neu et al., 1992). Consequently, in order to improve patient outcomes by reducing nosocomial infections, it has been widely recognized that sophisticated, active, and timely intrahospital surveillance is needed (Neu et al., 1992; Shlaes et al., 1997).

DMSS uses association rules to detect complex or unsuspected patterns in laboratory medicine data. DMSS resembles GermWatcher in that it uses data gathered in the analysis of cultures. However, in contrast to both CIDM and GermWatcher, DMSS is not constrained to searching for predefined patterns.

System overview:

- The system uses raw culture and patient demographics extracted from the laboratory information system.
- These data are cleaned, normalized, and divided into 1-month partitions (preprocessing).
- For each partition, frequent sets are discovered.
- Association rules are generated from frequent sets.
- The history, a database that contains association rules and partition-specific information, is updated and analyzed for patterns.
- The patterns are presented to the domain expert for evaluation.

DMSS has been applied to intensive care unit (Moser et al., 1999) and hospital-wide data sets (Brossette et al., in press). Example patterns from the analysis of inpatient data from the University of Alabama at Birmingham Hospital are given in the following table.

Example 1 shows that in March, the number of multidrug resistant nosocomial *Acinetobacter baumannii* [5] among all isolates [511] increased significantly compared to the previous 3 months. This finding was consistent with that of a traditional investigation.

Example 2 shows that the incidence of multidrug resistance in nosocomial *Klebsiella pneumoniae* increased significantly in January compared

Table 1 Examples of DMSS Alerts

No.	Surveillance Item (Denominator)		Outcome (Numerator)	Oct-96	Nov-96	Dec-96	Jan-97	Feb-97	Mar-97
		Association Rule (Alert)							
1	All Isolates	⇒	*Acinetobacter baumanii* Noso CAZ, PIP, TM, GM, AN, CIP, ATM, MZ, TIM, OFX, CTX, SxT			0/477	0/599	0/523	5/511
2	*Klebsiella pneumoniae* Noso	⇒	CTT, CAZ, CXM, CZ, PIP, SxT, CR, TM, GM, TIM, CRO	1/11	0/22	1/23	11/25		
3	*Streptococcus pneumoniae* NonNoso	⇒	E, P, CRO	1/6	0/9	0/9	4/9		

Note. Noso = nosocomial; NonNoso = community acquired.
Each antibiotic listed in an association is indicative of a resistant result, e.g., R~Antibiotic. AN = Amikacin; ATM = Aztreonam; CAZ = Ceftazidime; CIP = Ciprofloxacin; CR = Cephalothin; CRO = Ceftriaxone; CTT = Cefotetan; CTX = Cefotaxime; CXM = Cefuroxime; CZ = Cefazolin; E = Erythromycin; GM = Gentamicin; MZ = Mezlocillin; OFX = Ofloxacin; P = Penicillin; PIP = Piperacillin; SxT = Trimethoprim/Sulfmethoxazole; TIM = Ticarcillin/Clavulanic acid; TM = Tobramycin.

86

to the previous 3 months. This was not found by traditional surveillance methods.

Example 3 indicates that of the community acquired (nonnosocomial) *Streptococcus pneumoniae* isolated [9] there was an increase in the proportion expressing penicillin, ceftriaxone, and erythromycin resistance [4] in January compared to the previous 3 months. This finding is most relevant to the selection of empiric antimicrobial therapy for patients admitted with community-acquired pneumonia not recognized at the time by traditional methods.

DMSS represents a new type of exploratory data-mining system that efficiently identifies complex or unexpected and potentially interesting patterns in hospital infection control and public health surveillance data. As described by Dean and coworkers (1994), the ideal public health surveillance system of the future will include analysis tools that automatically identify, on different time and geographical scales, unusual and interesting patterns from time slices of raw data. Likewise, infection control systems of the future will require tools that recognize trends in nosocomial infection and antimicrobial resistance in an efficient and timely manner (Shlaes et al., 1997). The impact of DMSS on hospital patient outcomes awaits prospective implementation and evaluation currently in progress.

SUMMARY AND CONCLUSIONS

With the explosion in the volume of data, expanded database software capabilities, and rapid advances in the speed and storage capacity of hardware, there is an opportunity and a need to develop new tools for outcomes studies. The application of data mining to the domain of laboratory medicine is only in its infancy. The challenges laboratory medicine scientists face as stewards of the laboratory database are to assist in the development of data mining tools and to determine if they have the potential to affect laboratory or patient outcomes.

REFERENCES

Alnahi H, Alshawi S. Knowledge discovery in biomedical databases: A machine induction approach. *Computer Methods Prog. Biomed.* 1993;39:343–349.

Anand T, Kahn G. SPOTLIGHT: A data explanation system. *Proc. Eighth IEEE Conf. Applied AI*, pp. 2–8. IEEE Press, Piscataway, NJ, 1992.

Blanchard D. New watch. *AI Expert* 1994;7:3.

Brossette S, Sprague AP, Jones WT, Moser SA. A data mining system for infection control surveillance. *Methods Inform. Med.* (in press).

Brossette SE, Sprague AP, Hardin JM, Waites KB, Jones WT, Moser SA. Association rules and data mining in hospital infection control and public health surveillance. *J. Am. Med. Inform. Assoc.* 1998;5:373–381.

Burke JP, Classen DC, Pestotnik SL, Evans RS, Stevens LE. The HELP system and its application to infection control. *J. Hosp. Infec. Control* 1991;18(suppl. A): 424–431.

Dean AG, Fagan RF, Panter-Conner BJ. Computerizing public health surveillance systems. In: Teutsch SM, Churchill RE (eds.), *Principles and Practice of Public Health Surveillance,* pp. 200–217. Oxford University Press, New York, 1994.

Evans RS, Burke JP, Classen DC, Gardner RM, Menlove RL, Goodrich KM, Stevens LE, Pestotnik SL. Computerized identification of patients at high risk for hospital-acquired infection. *Am. J. Infec. Control* 1992;20:4–10.

Evans RS, Larsen RA, Burke JP, Gardner RM, Meier FA, Jacobson JA, Conti MT, Jacobson JT, Hulse RK. Computer surveillance of hospital-acquired infections and antibiotic use. *JAMA* 1986;256:1007–1011.

Fayyad UM, Piatetsky-Shapiro B, Smyth P, Uthurusamy R. From data mining to knowledge discovery: An overview. In: Fayyad UM, Piatesky-Shapiro G, Smyth P, Uthurusamy R (eds.*), Advances in Knowledge Discovery and Data Mining,* pp. 1–34. AAAI Press, Menlo Park, NJ, 1996.

Frawley WJ, Pietetsky-Shapiro G, Matheus C J. Knowledge discovery in databases: An overview. *AI Mag.* 1992;13(3):1445–1453.

Hall J, Mani G, Barr D. Applying computational intelligence to the investment process. In: *Anonymous Proceedings of CIFER-96: Computational Intelligence in Financial Engineering,* pp. 10–18. IEEE Press, Piscataway, NJ, 1996.

Hand D. Data mining: Statistics and more? *Am. Stat.* 1998;52:112–118.

Holfacker IL, Huynen MA, Stadler PF, Stolorz PE. Knowledge discovery in RNA sequence families of HIV using scalable computers. *Proc. Second Inter. Conf. Knowledge Discovery and Data Mining.* AAAI Press, Menlo Park, NJ, 1996.

IBM. Data mining: Advanced Scout [online]. IBM Website. 1995. http://www.research.ibm.com/scout/ Accessed 06/16/1999.

John GH. Enhancements to the data mining process. University of Michigan, Ann Arbor, Dissertation, 1997.

Kahn MG, Steib SA, Fraser VJ, Dunagan WC. An expert system for culture-based infection control surveillance. *Proc. Annu Symp. Computer Applications in Medical Care* 1993;171–175.

Kahn MG, Steib SA, Dunagan WC, Fraser VJ. Monitoring expert system performance using continuous user feedback. *J. Am. Med. Inform. Assoc.* 1996a;3: 216–223.

Kahn MG, Bailey TC, Steib SA, Fraser VJ, Dunagan WC. Statistical process control methods for expert system performance monitoring. *J. Am. Med. Inform. Assoc.* 1996b;3:258–269.

Matheus CJ, Piatesky-Shapiro G, McNeill D. Selecting and reporting what is interesting: The KEFIR application to health-care data. In: Fayyad UM, Piatesky-Shapiro G, Smyth P, Uthurusamy R (eds.*), Advances in Knowledge Discovery and Data Mining,* pp. 495–516. AAAI Press, Menlo Park, NJ, 1996.

McDonald JM, Brossette S, Moser SA. Pathology information systems: Data mining leads to knowledge discovery. *Arch. Pathol. Lab. Med.* 1998;122:409–411.

Moser SA, Jones WT, Brossette SE. Application of data mining to intensive care unit microbiologic data. *Emerg. Infec. Dis.* 1999;5(3):454–457.

Neu HC, Duma RJ, Jones RN, McGowan JEJ, O'Brien TF, Sabath LD, et al. Antibiotic resistance: Epidemiology and therapeutics. *Diagn. Microbiol. Infect. Dis.* 1992;2:53–60.

Prather JC, Lobach DF, Goodwin LK, Hales JW, Hage ML, Hammond WE. Medical data mining: Knowledge discovery in a clinical data warehouse. *Proc. AMIA Ann. Fall Symp.* 1997;101–105.

Rocha BH, Christenson JC, Pavia A, Evans RS, Gardner RM. Computerized detection of nosocomial infections in newborns. *Proc. Ann. Symp. Computer Applications in Medical Care* 1994;684–688.

Shek EC, Muntz RR, Mesrobian E, Ng K. Scalable exploratory data mining of distributed geoscientific data. *Proc. Second Int. Conf. Knowledge Discovery and Data Mining* 1996;32–37.

Shlaes DM, Gerding DN, John JFJ, Craig WA, Bornstein DL, Duncan RA, et al. Society for Healthcare Epidemiology of American and Infectious Diseases Society of American Joint Committee on the Prevention of Antimicrobial Resistance: Guidelines for the prevention of antimicrobial resistance in hospitals. *Clin. Infec. Dis.* 1997;25:584–599.

Tsai YS, King PH, Higgins MS, Pierce D, Patel NP. An expert-guided decision tree construction strategy: an application in knowledge discovery with medical databases. *Proc. AMIA Ann. Fall Symp.* 1997:208–212.

Tsumoto S, Ziarko W, Shan N, Tanaka H. Knowledge discovery in clinical databases based on variable precision rough set model. *Proc. Ann. Symp. Computer Applications in Medical Care* 1995:270–274.

Wong D, Jones WT, Brossette S, Hardin JM, Moser, SA. A strategy for geomedical surveillance using the Hawkeye knowledge discovery system. Gierl L, Cliff AD, Valleron AJ, Farrington P, Bull M. *Geomed '97.* Teubner Stuttgart, Leipzig, 1998:204–213.

Chapter 8

Outcomes-Based Decision Support: How to Link Laboratory Utilization to Clinical Endpoints

L. H. Bernstein

OVERVIEW AND PURPOSE

The laboratory historically produces good quality data, but the data have to be converted to useful information. Our most important product is information, not the generation of isolated unrelated tests. Our contribution to the medical enterprise will be assessed only in the context of the impact of our output on clinical services affected by direct care providers. We have the opportunity to align our activities with the medical enterprise through outcomes research. Outcomes research is now a critical activity focused on improving ends and means. Health-care providers have to use outcomes research to be competitive in a changed health-care landscape that is characterized by financial risk to provider organizations. This new environment is characterized by excess variation in use of medical procedures and technologies. There is medical as well as financial risk in all utilization decisions. The only way to evaluate these choices and their consequences is a structured quality management program with an outcomes research backbone (Speicher and Smith, 1983).

Risk adjustment is essential for examining the effects of treatments and comparing the outcomes of care across and even within populations. Risk adjustment as carried out using administrative databases relies on the interactive and additive associations between comorbidities and measured outcomes, such as, length of stay, readmissions, and cost of care (Iezzone, 1997). This approach is quite unsatisfactory for giving any insights into the relationships between the care process and the outcome measured. It explains no more than a third of the associated outcome. A better approach is the systematic capture of any explanatory data throughout the care process for use in risk adjustment. That is an approach that is used in acute care to stratify the sickest patients, such as using APACHE II or III, or injury severity score (ISS) (Iezzone, 1997). The approach may use clinical data, such as vital signs, and may be laboratory inclusive.

The use of the laboratory is especially appealing because it is readily available by linkage of the laboratory to clinical databases. The most common laboratory tests included are pCO_2, bicarbonate, potassium, albumin, hematocrit, and white cell count. Mozes et al. (1994) showed that patients could be classified into severity of illness groups using seven laboratory tests as well as by a clinical method. The clinical laboratory can become an architect of its future by having a leading role in guiding the use of its information product. I explore methods by which we can perform quality control on the information product of the laboratory, increasing the value of the reporting. The reader will have a better understanding of why we would want to pursue these approaches, gain some understanding of how and when to use them, and even discard a reluctance to get involved because of assumptions about the difficulties of the task.

THE CHALLENGE OF STUDY DESIGN FOR OUTCOMES RESEARCH

The NIH randomized prospective clinical trial (RPT) is outcome based, but can be very costly and produces limited conclusions. These studies require the definition of exclusion and inclusion criteria, the collection of data over a long period of time, and enough statistical power to determine significance. There is often no justification for carrying out the RPT outside of an academic setting, and it often requires multiple sites. It is used merely to eliminate an underlying systematic selection bias that can undermine the conclusions in testing a hypothesis. It requires a rigorous method of data collection using a case report format. The method of RPT can't eliminate the random unintended effects that occur in a clinical setting. It also can't answer questions about effects or hypotheses that are outside the study design. These effects are the basis for a notable discrepancy in effectiveness in a procedure, test, or method when introduced after efficacy has been shown. On the other hand, data collected by a case-study format can be done prospectively, and the results can be used with astounding benefit to the organization. This can be done again and again.

THE CHALLENGE OF CONVERTING DATA TO USEFUL INFORMATION

The laboratory is an environment dedicated to producing quality-controlled results used in patient care management. The output of the laboratory is the information component of its product and the decisions that flow from its activities. We are interested in influencing clinical decisions. These are associated with clinical assessments. They are tied to logical structures that are only partly captured by existing medical terminology. We are committed to examining the associations between the laboratory output and medical states. We can anticipate reporting significant associations to those who use the information. What we have become interested in is the continuous capture of data. It has to be sufficient for *measuring the information* and for measuring clinical endpoints. The data set is derived from data easily captured, preferably by an automated or partly automated method. This is examined by a variety of methods. The adequacy of and structure of the data support decisions that allow for improvement.

We first consider the problems of data definition and data collection, complexity of the process described affecting the data handling requirements, correlation between variables used and expected outcomes, methods of analysis, and costs of the method of control versus cost of process controlled.

OUTCOME RESEARCH USES A STRUCTURED DATA MATRIX

Outcome research in a production setting of health-care delivery can be described as a formal systematized approach to self-examination, learning, and improvement using data, analysis, models, and reevaluation. The process has the following components:

1. Defining disease or disease(s) of interest.
2. Defining all the variables that contribute to the description or diagnosis.
3. Defining other clinical states and treatments that may be associated with or have an effect on the first two items.
4. Defining changes in the first three items that are expected with improvement or decline of function in the clinical state(s).
5. The first four items make up the data set necessary to examine diseases and treatments by collecting data on the disease states and looking for association between the data and desired outcomes.
6. The data collected have value insofar as they contribute to the discrimination between disease states or treatment effects.
7. Data have little value insofar as they make no contribution to resolution of disease states or treatment effects.
8. The strength of data is in the ability to resolve uncertainty. We later show how we use the data better for certain questions by scaling the data.
9. There can be more than one outcome, and outcomes can be related.

A STATISTICAL FRAMEWORK AND BEYOND NORMALITY

Clinical chemistry has used statistics for statistical quality control. The confidence intervals generated by testing were based on an assumed normal distribution, and a willingness to ignore normal noise, which is medical. Galen and Gambino (1975; Krieg et al., 1983) and Martin et al. (1975) have taught that the test reference limits are decision values that result in assigned error rates. We are accustomed to using an assumed normal distribution and two standard deviations from the center as a reference (Martin et al., 1975). We really use the intersection of two curves to make a decision about a boundary choice, which is described in a 2-by-2 contingency table (Hayes, 1981; Selterman and Louis, 1992; Jekel et al., 1996b). Truth tables and contingency tables are two ways of formating the same data.

The contingency table has the format:

	FALSE/ABSENT	TRUE/PRESENT
FALSE/ABSENT		
TRUE/PRESENT		

The truth table format is:

FF
TF
FT
TT

This is a simple construct and is a building block for multivariable methods. If we then add another test, this adds a real element of dimensionality. Using contingency tables, one has to do two sets of cross tables of predictor(s) versus response(s). Then one can combine cross tables for a bivariate table versus a single dependent variable. There are very powerful tests that are used with the contingency table, such as, Fisher's exact test for 2-by-2 matrices with a total cell count of 100 or fewer (Jekel et al., 1996). In a truth table, one would list the classes that are unique sets in rows with their defining characteristic in the first column, and the second column would be their frequency count, as we later explore further. The outcome variable is depicted next with two tests as predictors, shown as the familiar separate "training," or dependent variable.

Classes	Features
Disease Absent	
1	00
2	01
3	10
4	11
Disease Present	
1	00
2	01
3	10
4	11

The use of a single test always has the problem of considerable noise, which is only resolved by providing sufficient information. The use of combinations of tests allows us to form a classification matrix, which we use to account for the variability explained. In all of the models we encounter there is a predictor or predictors and there is a dependent variable. The predictors are associated with the outcome or dependent variable through an association function. The strength of the association is tested, and the partial contribution of each test or predictor is usually measured by the association function. The methods for examining the relationship of laboratory data to patient outcomes can be described in three main approaches: linear and generalized regression models for continuous variables with ordinary least squares estimates (Jekel et al., 1996; Draper and Smith, 1981); logistic regression for dichotomous variables; and log-linear models. The last includes a graphical ordinal model using maximal likelihood estimation for polytomous variables, having more than two values (as opposed to dichotomous) (Magidson, 1995, 1996). Kooperberg, Bose, and Stone (1997) describe the problem of fitting a regression model to data involving a multivalued response variable and one or more predictors. Outside of these is a method of forming a continuous learning matrix, which can be combined with the last method (Rypka, 1992). Linear regression has problems when the dependent variable is dichotomous because the residuals don't have constant variance, standard errors of the regression coefficients are wrong, and the R^2 measure is problematic. These problems are overcome using classification methods and universal regression (Magidson, 1995, 1996). We next further examine these concepts.

WHAT ARE DATA?

We want to consider two types of data. Data that are event associated, such as clinical characteristics, morbidities, disease states, are ordinal. Ordinal data are not necessarily binary and can be scaled to levels greater than 2 (yes versus no). When clinical variables are scaled to other than binary choices the possibilities for resolving uncertainty may be improved when the variable is used in combination with other variables. This is not just a way of creating "fuzzy sets," or grades of uncertainty. There is no basis for classifying data using a single classifier. The use of at least two variables permits the formation of four sets of binary combinations from two. The four classes can be assessed for an association with a dependent variable. The main problem with this type of data is inaccuracy in its use for classification because clinical criteria can be too inconsistent. Then it might be inadequate for assessing severity or change, and inconsistencies may be found when using the data to form a classification.

An example of this is the description of a pain, which may be stabbing, tearing, boring. This description can be extremely difficult because a patient may present without pain, or the patient may present with different degrees of in addition to different qualities of pain, e.g., the intensity and other features of the pain, its location, or changes in the pain over time. In forming a diagnostic classification using this data, it is necessary to examine combinations of these features and determine the probabilities of the relation of the feature combinations to disease states. It is also necessary to keep in mind that the probabilities for rule-in and rule-out can be treated as separate problems. Problems may arise in forming a classification because of inadequacy of the variables used, and it may suffer from absence of sufficient and adequate features. In examining this type of data we are also more concerned with the frequency of alternative descriptions compared to the likelihood of the predicted event.

The use of clinical data is more limited than the ways in which we can analyze continuous data. Continuous data has a measure of magnitude, and it also can be scaled to be used in a classification. Continuous data has an advantage over descriptive data because it has information that can be used for assessing severity or intensity, and is well suited for assessing change. Continuous data are good for looking at dose-response effects. However, the interest in using continuous variables is often to ascertain whether an effect is absent, small, moderate, large, or very large. In this example, then, the data are associated with values of the variable to binary or higher order outcomes. The data can be scaled, thereby converting the data to an ordinal response. We later examine methods in which we convert continuous data to an ordinal response when classifying data to examine associations between treatments and effects.

DEFINING THE OUTCOME

A test can only be described as effective with respect to an outcome definition. The critical issue for defining what is a good test or descriptor compared with its alternative is in determining the endpoint(s). Much of the disciplinary focus is on the value of a single class of observations. In the case of chest pain, it may be the characteristics of the pain, electrocardiographic (ECG) pattern, or serum level of a cardiac-specific enzyme or protein. This gets back to the World Health Organization (WHO) criteria, which themselves need modification, but which recognize more than a single criterion for acute myocardial infarction (AMI). These tests are compared with respect to their likelihood of a positive result with or in absence of disease. But what is the reference point for comparing the result with disease? The WHO criteria have not been sufficient to deal with a class of unstable angina (UA) that has features more like AMI than UA. The designation of "gold standard" is derivative of a univariate model in which a test is selected based on comparison with a chosen "reference standard" as a supervisory classifier. In this case, the ECG based on ST elevation, known to be insensitive, is the "gold standard" for AMI classification.

An alternative "reference standard" is a classification model that reflects the best estimate of uncertainty in the data. It is only possible because of autocorrelation in the data. Autocorrelation means that variables in a data set are associated and can be used to form a crosstable. Any classification model is constructed based on the assumption that the data (clinical and other types) form a self-classifying matrix with different levels of uncertainty in the variable combinations describing each patient. If the information that is used to classify is poor, then the classification uncertainty is very high. The effect of this is that the combination of features used to describe and classify has a high level of uncertainty, does not resolve uncertainty, and is at maximum entropy. It is possible to eliminate from the "reference matrix" descriptors that make no contribution to resolving uncertainty.

DATA TO OUTCOMES

Consider a way to visualize data and outcomes. More than one outcome is possible and they may be related. All outcomes are products of and associated with data elements that are inputs. One can conceptualize data in the framework of observations and conclusions. Observations may be listed in one column while conclusions are listed in the other. This means that there are likely to be more observations than conclusions. But there has to be an association between the data on the left and the conclusions on the right. This method is a functional way of working with aggregate as well as individual data. It is a nice way to summarize a single patient. The column on the left we consider to be usable data, and that on the right is tag along, but it actually represents hypotheses generated by the data.

DATA PROPERTIES

It is important to consider that the data have an additional property not inherent in the observation of a single event. The data may change over two or more observations, whether the data are continuous or ordinal in expression. This is extremely important because the observation of the same variable over time, being stochastic, results in different variables having the same name identified only by difference in time or difference in trajectory (changed or not changed). This means that constructing a record of effects and treatments in the course of a patient's illness (acute or chronic) requires that all of the relevant data has to be captured, including repetitive data elements that have to be mapped into diagnoses, morbidities, and treatment responses. We also consider that features on the left may map into more than one (from a variety) of the response variables on the right. The left-hand and right-hand mapping lead to the view that the left-hand mapping into the right hand is a set of logical propositions.

We are particularly interested in laboratory data because the laboratory generates the largest part of the computerized record used by physicians for medical decisions. In fact, data capture of clinical variables is inadequate to describe as a significant feature of the computerized medical record. On the other hand, the interpretation of clinical data is an essential part of the practice of medicine. There can be no quality measurement without the systematic capture and evaluation of such information. Therefore, we first consider the features of the clinical data.

DATABASE DEFINITION

The creation of and wide experience with Lotus and Excel has taught many of us how to look at data structure in a simple way. The patients are in rows and each variable is a column. The analysis of data structures goes to the analysis of matrices and maybe of arrays. The manipulation of the data is carried out by a function. Functions exist in a spreadsheet, and they are more extensive in statistical programs. The following definitions are useful:

Data: Numbers, or letters and symbols that a function operates on.

Function: List of instructions for performing a task.

Variable: Storage place for data. The data can be numerical and continuous, categorical, or ordinal.

Scalar: Single number.

Vector: A sequence of numbers.

Matrix: A table of data. The two dimensions are rows and columns.

Array: A table of more than two dimensions. Rows and columns are separated by spaces. The number of dimensions is defined. In the example of chest pain and cardiac markers, the creatine kinase isoenzyme MB (CK-MB) may be defined as a separate variable for each time, but the time of sampling is linked to the CK-MB. The time of sampling can be used to create an n-dimensional array with the variables being the same across different time dimensions. In this case, there are n time dimensions for each CK-MB value.

AN EXAMPLE OF A CLINICAL DATA STRUCTURE

The presentation of the patient with acute onset of chest discomfort is a perfect example. Features that describe the characteristics of the chest pain include time of onset, location, duration, relief by nitrates, radiation, quality (pressing, crushing; *not* dull, penetrating, sharp, tearing), compared to previous chest pain. There are patient characteristics in addition to the characteristics of the chest pain, such as previous acute myocardial infarct, history of coronary vascular disease, and risk factors associated with coronary vascular disease. There are also physiological features that may describe the patient, such as EKG changes characteristic of AMI, dyspnea and rales at the lung bases, and ability to carry out physical activity (the basis for a stress exercise test).

The diagnosis of acute myocardial infarction (AMI) can't be made independently of the data used to classify patients. The accuracy of diagnosis is largely dependent on the features of the data set (Rypka, 1992) that allow the formation of classes that reduce the classification uncertainty. The Goldman algorithm (Goldman et al., 1982, 1988) is a set of criteria that identifies the likelihood of AMI in patients presenting to the emergency department with symptoms suggestive of AMI. In order to examine the effectiveness of the algorithm, one has to establish the order of contribution of the clinical criteria and laboratory tests to the diagnosis of AMI.

A standard questionnaire has been used prospectively to obtain history from all patients and, together with the admission electrocardiogram for each patient, evaluated by the Goldman algorithm. The decision about whether the patient has AMI or not is validated using three standards. These are: (1) characteristic evolution of isoenzyme CK-MB and LD1 obtained at 12 hours after admission (this standard will be supplanted by the troponins T and I); (2) new Q waves of at least 0.04 sec duration and at least a 25% decrease in the amplitude of the following R wave as compared with that of the EKG obtained in the emergency room; and (3) sudden unexplained death within 24 hours. Any statistical algorithm and clinical convention are both data dependent. The determination of whether there is AMI or not is carried out prospectively and independently of the classification algorithm.

The features described are all data elements, and some of them can change (ST segment) in a few hours. Of course, an association model that captures the expected change more likely with a "syndromic" combination of expected data elements can examine the likelihood of change in a few hours. At this point, I have not brought into the context the appearance and disappearance of an enzyme (CK, LD) or protein (troponin T or I) in serum after the onset of chest pain. In the case of creatine kinase isoenzyme MB, there is a characteristic evolution that is useful for classifying patients and for assessing their prognosis. From a classical perspective, these are not elevated early enough in the time course of AMI to be useful when patients present within less than 4 hours after the onset of chest pain. Although we have actually verified this, one has a sense that nonclassical presentation has an unlikely association with elevated serum laboratory markers of myocardial injury later, and will be unlikely to prove out to be AMI. On the other hand, the presence of crushing pain for 3 hours, radiation to the left arm, unrelieved by nitrates, and 2 mm ST elevation on EKG leaves little uncertainty about what is expected in the CK-MB or other markers of myocardial damage. Of course, an intermediate course is atypical presentation, perhaps T-wave inversion or ST-T depression, which requires the laboratory to resolve uncertainty. In the emergency department (ED) setting, patients have to be assessed as to low and high risk for AMI so that a decision can be made about discharge, use of an ED holding area, and admission to a CCU or monitored bed.

These features, clinical, laboratory, and other, can be captured systematically in a continuous learning matrix. The features are descriptor variables arranged in columns and the patients are in rows. Each patient is a statement described by the features in a line of a truth table. Eugene Rypka has described how this learning matrix learns, by rearrangement of the variables in the order of the information supplied to resolve uncertainty (Rypka, 1992). This is calculated by summing the values of the scaled variables. The scaled variables are rearranged in descending order. The patients are rearranged in rows so that they form distinctive classes with repeating patterns of the variable combinations. These patterns occur with an expected frequency, and they map into all of the diseases and morbidities that can be observed.

Another example that requires the use of both clinical and laboratory features (not necessarily at the same time) is the identification of patients with serious protein-energy malnutrition (with or without other nutritional deficits) (Shaw-Stiffel et al., 1993). Increasingly, the nursing service is assigned to carry out the initial evaluation using subjective risk factor identification. This leads to a nutritional evaluation. Risk factors that are identified include: involuntary weight loss in excess of 10% of usual weight, inability or unwillingness to take in food, dementia, diarrhea and/or vomiting, disease or condition affecting absorption or utilization of food (e.g., Crohn's disease), major trauma, or major surgery associated with hypermetabolism. A truth table has to include these as data elements. Laboratory data include albumin, cholesterol, transferrin, and prealbumin. Other tests are of interest if a patient receives intravenous nutrition. Outcome variables that may be viewed as important data include major complications (sepsis, wound dehiscence, pneumonia, ventilator dependency, ARDS/SIDS, renal failure, death), and minor complications (wound site infection, atalectasis, pulmonary edema, urinary tract infection, and decubitus). One has to also capture interventions: $\geq 60\%$ of needs met, Respiratory Therapy assessment, type of feeding, time to intervention, number of interventions, return to activities of daily living, and failure to implement recommendations.

GOLD STANDARD(S)

It is usually necessary in introducing a diagnostic method to compare it against a "gold standard" or supervisory classification, against which all methods are compared. This is increasingly problematic as illustrated by the observation of elevated cardiac troponin T (cTnT) with negative CK-MB in patients with ischemic coronary syndromes and risk of subsequent death or cardiac event. The usual 2-by-2 table for disease present or absent versus test positive or negative is not a representation that accounts for all of the clinical events. Assigning the correct diagnosis of AMI without using isoenzymes has become impossible whenever chest pain is atypical and EKG changes are equivocal. Consequently, the diagnosis of AMI can't be made independently of the data used to classify patients, and a gold standard is a fluid reference. The accuracy of diagnosis is largely dependent on the features of the data set that allow the formation of classes that reduce the classification uncertainty. Using methods that classify the data and increasing the information content of the data should be particularly valuable in studying the ischemic coronary syndromes, including non-Q-wave AMI.

METHODS FOR DATA ANALYSIS IN OUTCOMES EVALUATION

The most commonly used methods are univariate analysis of the means, the median, standard deviation, and variance. For example, given an exposure and the comparison of patients who become infected or remain uninfected, the means of the populations are determined. A histogram describes the frequency of infected versus not infected. If the question is infection rate associated with a particular procedure versus another, then the means or medians of the infection rates are compared (*t*-test) or the frequencies are compared in a cross-tabulation with a chi-square test of whether they are the same or different.

Linear regression methods. Linear regression explores the fit of a line to a set of data represented by a response variable and a predictor variable. The response (predicted) variable may be continuous or ordinal, but the predictor variable is usually continuous. When the response (predicted) variable is ordinal, the linear model breaks down to a one-way analysis of variance (ANOVA) model. When a continuous variable is fitted to a single predictor, the simple linear regression is expressed by the equation:

$$Y = a + bX$$

where a is the Y intercept, b is the slope of the regression line, and a or b is derived from the method of ordinary least squares (OLS).

The method of OLS uses the *F*-test for the mean squared errors and requires the assumption of normality of the errors. The measure of fit is R^2. The use of multiple variables in the regression to predict another variable is termed a multiple regression model. The multiple regression model has to meet the assumptions that the fit is linear, the predictors are independent and have no collinearity, and the errors have a constant variance and are uncorrelated across observations.

Logistic regression. The linear regression model is extended when the predictor variables are coded 0,1 and the response is a probability from 0 to 1. In the case of logistic regression the response variable is two-valued or binary.

"Group-based reference."   We have shown that there is no justifiable definition of normal reference in a population defined by a single attribute (or test) without referring to a supervisory classification (Rudolph et al., 1988). Such an approach requires validation by use of an ROC curve. This condition is eliminated by treating diagnostic tests as a message transmission and the provision of information as reduction of uncertainty (Rudolph et al., 1988; Rypka, 1992).

We described an information-based model (Rudolph et al., 1988) in which the disease and normal reference populations are complementary subsets, one of which has information, the other of which is empty (has no information). These groups can be differentiated even without a supervisory classification by using a defining set of characteristics (tests) which, when combined, reduce the uncertainty in the data relation. In the case of acute myocardial infarction, for example, CK-MB, LD1, and %LD1 results, classified as positive (1) or negative (0), may be used to form a three-letter word (e.g., 101). The assignment of these words to patients clusters them into any of eight groups (000, 001, 010, 100, 111, 110, 011, 101), allowing assignment to either AMI or non-AMI with less than 1% misclassification error based on the occurrence of at least two positive results.

In examining the general data set for endogenous information, we find critical decision limits that produce binary pattern classes allowing minimum error assignment to a reference classification. We find these decision limits by examining the entropy of the data relations and take the frequency distribution and probabilities of the binary classes formed using incremented values assigned to each variable paired with the median or optimum value of the other variables. The maximum entropy of the data is found by destroying the information from the correlation in the data by randomizing the variables and taking the frequency distribution and probabilities of the binary classes produced. The maximum entropy distribution of a binary pattern is not flat but has a greater frequency of all positive and all negative patterns.

To examine the information characteristics of each variable, we plot entropy as a function of decision level. For each binary decision point, the entropy of the probability distribution of the binary pattern classes is compared to that obtained using a data matrix in which the information is destroyed. The point of maximum effective information is that which relieves the most uncertainty in the database and yields the fewest errors in discrimination.

MINIMUM FEATURES SET AND ATTRIBUTE EXTRACTION

A primary database is expressed in a matrix format, with each patient a row and each attribute characteristic or predicate variable a column. Rypka (1992) describes a method for extracting features over all of the elements in a paired comparison such that the minimum features can be found that separate all possible pairs of elements. This pattern arrangement is represented in the truth table.

It is expected that in most data sets there are more features than the theoretical number in the matrix for N elements or events. One can determine how far the real is from the theoretical by extracting the theoretical minimum number of features,

$$h = \log_R N.$$

Whatever h is, for each combination, h features will be extracted. If h (features) = 3, N (diseases) = 8, and the number of predicate variables is 32, we expect to define the fewest predicate variables (Rudolph et al., 1988) taken three at a time that maximize the separation of eight diseases. This is expressed by the equation for s, separation:

$$s = \frac{1}{2} [N^2 - (n_{111}^2 + n_{110}^2 + n_{101}^2 + n_{100}^2 + n_{011}^2 + n_{010}^2 + \cdots)]$$

The combination of features that maximizes s minimizes entropy. The process of maximizing information content and optimizing separation is tied to uncertainty in information theory. Information is the uncertainty that is resolved by the data.

Neural network and preprocessing.   We cluster using the geometrical (Euclidean) distance between two points in n-dimensional space, formed by n variables. Since this distance assumes compatibility of different variables, the values of all input variables are linearly transformed (scaled) to the range from 0 to 1. For readers accustomed to classical statistics, the neural network technique can be viewed as an extension of multivariate regression analyses with such new features as nonlinearity and ability to process categorical data. The latter refers to the output variable allowing a classification into two (in case of binary output) or more classes.

The neural network is an acyclic directed graph with input and output nodes corresponding respectively to input and output variables. There are also "intermediate" nodes, comprising so-called "hidden" layers. Each node n_i is assigned the value x_i that has been evaluated by the node's "processing" element, acting as a nonlinear function of the weighted sum of values x_h of nodes n_h, connected with n_i by directed edges (n_h, n_i):

$$x_i = f(w_{h(1),i}x_{h(1)} + w_{h(2),i}x_{h(2)} + \cdots + w_{h(k),i}x_{h(k)})$$

where x_h is the value in node n_h and $w_{h,i}$ is the "weight" of the edge (n_h, n_i). In our research we used the standard function f(x), "sigmoid," defined as $f(x) = 1/[1 + \exp(-x)]$. This function is suitable for categorical output and allows for using an efficient back-propagation algorithm for calculating the optimal values of weights, providing the best fit for learning set of data, and eventually the most accurate classification.

We implemented the proposed algorithm for diagnosis of AMI. All the calculations were performed on IBM-compatible 486DX-33 computer, using the authors' (I. Mayzlin and L. Bernstein) unique Maynet software running in MS-DOS. First, using the automatic random extraction procedure, the initial data set is partitioned into two sets—training and testing. This randomization also determines the size of these sets after the program is instructed to partition into two approximately equal groups.

The main process consists of three successive steps:

1. Clustering performed on training data set.
2. Neural network's training on clusters from previous step.
3. Classifier's accuracy evaluation on testing data.

The classifier in this research is the neural network, created on step 2, with output in the range [0,1], that provides binary result (1 for AMI, 0 for not AMI), using decision point 0.5.

Graphical Ordinal Logit Display.   Jay Magidson (Statistical Innovations, Belmont, MA) (Littenberg and Moses, 1993; Qu and Hagdu, 1998) has developed a polytomous approach to probability estimation using ordinal variables whereby quantitative scores may or may not be assigned to the categories, but category spacing is assumed to exist. The method assumes a monotonic relationship and uses maximum likelihood estimation (Haberman, 1995). It uses a log odds model fit, and the odds ratio is obtained from the log(odds ratio). In the linear probability model, the coefficients (b_i) are partial correlation coefficients. In the logit model the coefficients are partial log(odds ratio). The results are expressed graphically in a GOLDminer (graphical ordinal logit display) interface. The method is polytomous because the outcome can have more than one predictor variable.

CASE STUDY 1. EVALUATING A NEW TEST FOR PRETERM LABOR

Fetal fibronectin is a new test for preterm labor that is based on measuring a protein secreted by chorionic trophoblasts present in low concentrations in maternal serum that increases as a result of membrane compromise from 24 to 35 weeks gestation. A study of 192 women with possible preterm labor (PTL) and cervical dilation <3 cm showed the test to predict delivery within 7 days, with sensitivity 0.93, specificity 0.82, positive predictive value 0.29, and negative predictive value 0.99. One can take the equations and calculate from them the following: true positive, 13; false positive, 32; true negative, 146; false negative, 1. The 2-by-2 table that describes the data is as follows:

	Observed Counts	
	PTL(−)	PTL(+)
FFN(−)	146	1
FFN(+)	32	13

The observed probabilities are obtained by summing the FFN frequencies across the rows and taking the ratio of each cell to its corresponding sum. Thus, the probability for FFN(−), PTL(−) = 146/146 + 1 = 0.99, and that for FFN(+), PTL(−) = 0.71. In this case we are interested in the absence of labor as the desired effect, and the fetal fibronectin test as the treatment. One is less interested in this case in the outcome preterm labor using the FFN test. The probability for FFN(−), PTL(+) = 1/147 = 0.01, using the negative test counts as a control row. This probability is recognized as the predictive value of a negative FFN. The FFN(+), PTL(+) = 0.29. The probability of the first row may be referred to as P_c, and of the second as P_t. The probabilities across the rows add to 1.

	Observed Probabilities		
	PTL(−)	PTL(+)	y-ref
FFN(−)	0.99	0.01	29.97
FFN(+)	0.71	0.29	101.52

Given the probabilities, we can calculate the corresponding odds o for any p using the following calculation:

$$o = p/(1 − p)$$

The odds in favor of an event is expressed as o, but the odds against it is o^{-1}. In the example, FFN(+) produces odds against PTL, so FFN(+), PTL(−) gives $o^{-1} = p/(1 − p)$. An observed probability is not necessarily the same as an expected probability. A probability is adjusted when some evidence is introduced to change our estimation of the probability. The probability before is called "prior probability," and the new probability is called "posterior probability," or "estimated probability." There is also a corresponding "prior odds" and "posterior odds." The ratio between these is the adjustment introduced by the new evidence. This is referred to as a Bayes factor. The adjustment is a calculation from probability densities.

A table of the observed odds from the ones just given is calculated from the counts directly by taking the results of the first column and dividing by the corresponding row counts in the second column (Selterman and Louis, 1992). Therefore, the odds for FFN(−), PTL(−) and FFN(+), PTL(−) are the counts of each, divided by the counts for FFN(−), PTL(+) and FFN(+), PTL(+). These are 146 and 2.46, respectively.

	Observed Odds	
	PTL(−)	**PTL(+)**
FFN(−)	146	1
FFN(+)	2.46	1

The Pearson chi-square is 40.555 for the 2-by-2 frequency table of fibronectin versus preterm labor (using SPSS or SYSTAT software). The expected odds ratio for fibronectin 0/1 is 59.313. The expected counts from the chi-square adjustment are:

	Expected Counts	
	PTL(−)	**PTL(+)**
FFN(−)	136.3	10.7
FFN(+)	41.7	3.3

We can calculate the expected counts for each cell. It is important to realize that for a 2-by-2 table the cells are determined by the row and column totals. We are testing whether there is significant difference between the cell counts and the expected cell counts. The formula for calculating the expected counts for each cell is:

(Row count) ×(column count)/total count

The expected counts for the top left cell, then, is $178 \times 147/192 = 136.3$. The same calculation is carried out on the remaining cells. The assumptions in the chi-square test may be invalid for a 2-by-2 table in which the cell count for any cell is less than 5. For a row by column table that is more than 2-by-2 cells, 20% of the counts are expected to be less than 5. A contingency table can be compressed to reduce the number of columns.

In this simple example, the 2-by-2 contingency table is tested by Fisher's exact test under the assumption that the odds ratio is 1. The row and column totals are held fixed, and the probability of the counts is compared with the expected counts under a hypothesis of independence. A more conservative calculation of the chi-square called the Yates correction is used for small sample studies to correct for continuity. The Pearson chi-square, used more often, is an approximation of the chi-square distribution. In this case, the differences between observed and the expected counts are used to calculate the chi-square (Selterman and Louis, 1992):

$$\text{Chi square} = \text{SUM} \frac{(\text{observed count} - \text{expected count})^2}{\text{expected count}}$$

One can calculate the expected odds using the information from the expected frequencies in the table above. The expected odds and expected odds ratios are calculated using the GOLDminer software. The expected baseline odds ratios are calculated by dividing each expected odds (provided) by the corresponding baseline odds associated with the given x-reference category.

The adjusted baseline odds are calculated by dividing each estimated observed count by the corresponding base count associated with the outcome base or reference category. These are based on using the derived base reference hidden from view. The odds against PTL given FFN($-$) is $146/101.52 = 1.438$, and for PTL given FFN($-$) is $1/101.52 = 0.01$. The odds against PTL given FFN($+$) is $32/29.97 = 1.068$, and the odds for PTL given FFN($+$) is $13/29.97 = 0.434$.

	Expected Odds		
	PTL($-$)	**PTL($+$)**	**y-ref**
FFN($-$)	1.438	0.01	1
FFN($+$)	1.068	0.434	1
x-ref	1.34	0.024	

The odds ratio is obtained by dividing the odds for the row used to demonstrate no effect, in this case FFN($-$), by the row with the effect, FFN($+$). Using the observed odds ratios of 146 and 2.46, the calculated odds ratio is 59.31. An odds ratio of 1 indicates independence of the treatment and the outcome, or a measure of no effect. An odds ratio that is less than or greater than 1 is a measure of the degree of dependence between the categorical variables.

	Expected Odds Ratio		
	PTL($-$)	**PTL($+$)**	**y-ref**
FFN($-$)	1.072	0.412	1
FFN($+$)	0.796	18.146	1
x-ref	1	1	

CASE STUDY 2. CARDIAC DIAGNOSIS AND A SELF-CLASSIFYING MATRIX

We compared the Goldman algorithm (Goldman et al., 1982, 1988) with total creatine kinase (CK) and CK-MB isoenzyme serially measured in serum at the time of admission and every 4 hours for 12 or 16 hours thereafter, and lactate dehydrogenase (LD) and the LD isoenzyme-1 at 12 hours after first sample. We thereby confirmed the effectiveness of the algorithm and could establish the order of contribution of the clinical criteria and laboratory tests to the diagnosis of AMI. The algorithm was demonstrated to be effective for emergency room triage with a specificity of 75% or greater for reducing admission of nonacute myocardial infarct (AMI) patients by 11.5%. The study allowed us to classify patients into AMI and non-AMI based on the amount of uncertainty in the clinical and laboratory data using the method of "group-based" reference (Rudolph et al., 1988). The method determines decision limits from the redundancy in the data, finding the value that produces fewest classification errors (Rudolph et al., 1988).

The LD1 12 hours, CK-MB 12 hours, CK-MB 8 hours, and %LD1 were the highest ranked tests for AMI classification. The Goldman algorithm with %LD1 was critical with equivocal patterns. The LD1/total LD was particularly important in non-Q-wave AMI, and it is the test best correlated with the algorithm. The study identified the need for a second stage of diagnosis/prediction beyond the Goldman algorithm using the laboratory.

PATIENT SELECTION

We carried out a prospective study on 200 patients admitted to the CCU with the primary diagnosis likelihood of AMI from the attending staff, and data was complete for 155 of these. We did not include patients seen in the emergency department (ED) and not admitted to the CCU since the Goldman algorithm was administered post hoc. The remaining 333 patients (62.5%) who did not qualify for the study had a variety of admitting diagnoses including unstable angina and congestive heart failure with or without AMI and arrhythmias that qualified them for placement in the CCU. The criteria for inclusion were primary diagnosis at admission of likely AMI; likely AMI the cause for admission to CCU; and no coexisting diagnosis that would warrant admission to the CCU. The criteria for exclusion were: admission for elective procedures; cardiac enzymes known prior to triage to CCU; triage decision aided by echocardiogram for wall motion abnormality; and admission for indications other than AMI evaluation.

The statistical algorithm and clinical convention are both data dependent. The determination of whether there was AMI or not was carried out prospectively and independently of the classification algorithm. It was recorded as a separate feature for comparison with the classified data. Most important about the method is the ability to determine optimum decision points for mapping the data into the independently determined diagnosis of AMI or not without prior reference to the diagnosis. LD1 was *only* taken at 12 hours after admission. The data were sufficient for statistical evaluation based on availability of LD1 for 155 of the 200 patients.

The optimum medical decision cutoffs were assigned using the method of group-based reference as determined using CK-MB, LD1, and LD1/total LD (percent LD1) by the method of Rudolph et al. (1988) (group-based reference).

CONSTRUCTION OF TRUTH TABLE

Clinical criteria	Scaling
1. ST elevation or Q-waves, 2 or more leads	0, 1
2. Chest pain began ≥48 hours ago	0, 1
3. ST-T changes	0, 1
4. History of angina or AMI	0, 1
5. Radiates to neck, left shoulder or left arm	0, 1
6. Longest ≥1 hour	0, 1
7. Age ≥40	0, 1
8. Worse than usual angina or same as earlier MI	0, 1
9. Reproduced by palpation	0, 1
10. Radiates to back, abdomen, legs	0, 1
11. Stabbing	0, 1

Laboratory criteria	Scaling		
	0	1	2
CK: 12-17 hours	<151 U/L	151–250 U/L	>250 U/L
CK-MB: 18-23 hours	negative	positive	
Total LD, 12 hours	<541 U/L	>540 U/L	
LD1	<200 U/L	200–299 U/L	>299 U/L
LD1/tLD (%)	<28%	29-31%	≥32%

The Goldman algorithm, its component criteria, and creatine kinase and lactate dehydrogenase and the isoenzymes of these taken at different times are used to classify patients with the tests from most to least important in classifying the data taken in descending order. The classification is compared with the rule-in diagnosis, taking into consideration that the Goldman algorithm is optimized for rule-out AMI.

We have shown that there is no justifiable definition of normal reference in a population defined by a single attribute (or test) without referring to a supervisory classification (Rudolph et al., 1988). Such an approach requires validation by use of a receiver operator characteristic (ROC) curve. This condition is eliminated by treating diagnostic tests as a message transmission and the provision of information as reduction of uncertainty

(Rudolph et al., 1988). The advantage of this is independence from any assumption about the nature and distribution of the data, and elimination of the defining set (Rudolph et al., 1988). The process of maximizing information content and optimizing separation is tied to uncertainty in information theory (Rypka, 1992). I show a plot (Figure 1) of CK-MB values on the x-axis versus information added (bits) and a paired comparison (Table 1) of cardiac troponin T and CK-MB with their binary patterns to demonstrate the entropy decision value concept.

Table 2 shows the frequencies of AMI in three groups of patients: AMI, equivocal, and non-AMI, based on CK, CK-MB, LD1, %LD1, and the Goldman chest pain algorithm. The Goldman algorithm was effective for emergency department triage of the chest pain patients (excluding patients admitted to CCU from ED for other reasons), identifying which CCU admissions were likely to have acute AMIs (sensitivity 99.5%, specificity 43%). The CK-MB is most discriminatory at 8 and 12 hours. The first four tests to classify in order are LD1, CK-MB 12h, CK-MB 8h, and %LD1. The Goldman algorithm is last.

The proportion of unequivocal AMI, equivocal, and non-AMI is 29.9%, 22.7%, and 47.4% (Table 2). The likelihood of AMI decreases: 100%, 86.4%, and 32.6%. The importance of the Goldman algorithm is in groups 2 and 3. There was a 72.7% frequency of LD1 and %LD1 with a rule-in AMI by the Goldman algorithm in the second group (equivocal), but the CK-MB added only one additional case. There was a 13% frequency of positive %LD1 in the third (non-AMI) group and 28.3% positive %LD1 with a rule-in AMI with a rule-in AMI diagnosis.

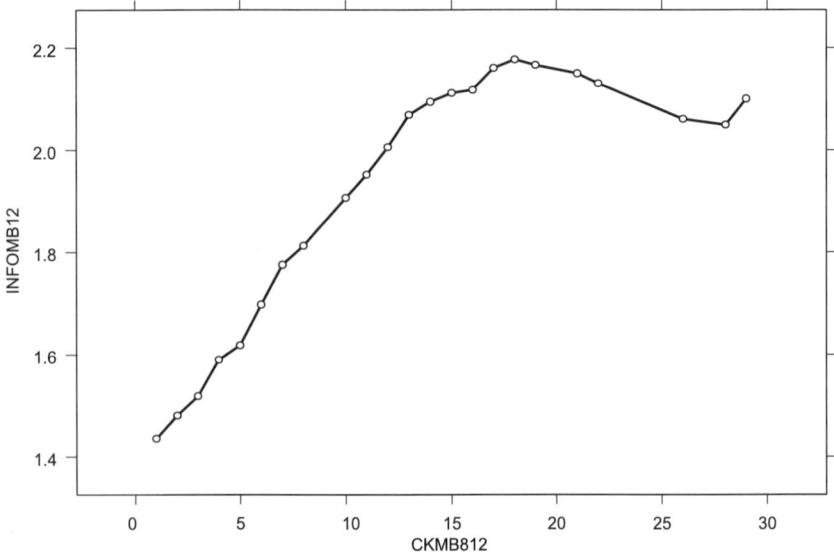

Figure 1 CK-MB values versus effective Information (bits).

Table 1   Paired Comparisons of cTnT and CK-MB With Combinatorial Classes

cTnT (ng/ml)	CK-MB (U/L)	PATTERN
0	5	0
0	9	0
0	4	0
0	13	0
0	4	0
0.01	1	0
0.01	4	0
0.01	12	0
0.02	12	0
0.02	7	0
0.02	7	0
0.03	16	0
0.03	14	0
0.03	8	0
0.04	10	0
0.05	8	0
0.05	8	0
0.05	6	0
0.06	15	0
0.07	13	0
0.08	7	0
0.08	10	0
0.09	15	0
0.10	9	0
0.11	7	0
0.11	7	0
0.12	25	11
0.14	12	10
0.14	12	10
0.15	3	10
0.16	158	11
0.16	33	11
0.16	23	11
0.18	1	10
0.18	46	11

Table 3 is a cross-tabulation from the data. The finding of a negative Goldman test is strongly associated with not AMI, but the patients without AMI may have a positive Goldman test.

The Goldman algorithm has similar sensitivity to the LD1/LD (%LD1) but can be used 12 hours sooner. The greatest value of LD1/LD (%LD1) is in the examination of non-Q-wave AMI, which accounts for 25.5% of the study population. Percent LD1 with ST-T changes without Q-waves was

Table 2   Frequency of AMI in Classes Defined by Classifiers

Group	Percent	Frequency AMI	Defining features
1	29.9	1.000	LD1, CK-MB 12h, 8h, %LD1
2	22.7	0.864	LD1, %LD1, Goldman
3	47.4	0.326	%LD1, Goldman

56.4%, ST-T changes without %LD1 occurred in 28.2%, and %LD1 with no ST-T changes indicated AMI in 15.4% of these patients. Percent LD1 was increased at 12 hours in 74% and CK-MB was increased at 8 hours in 71.8% of non-Q wave AMIs. 26 (66.7%) of the non-Q-wave patients had increased %LD1 and LD1, but only 18 (46.1%) had increased %LD1 and CK-MB.

The value of the CK-MB 8 hrs and LD1/LD (%) is to provide missing information to resolve uncertainty when the GOLDMAN is positive. The entropy decision limits define the confidence intervals shown in Table 4 in the Goldman test positive group. Table 5 shows how each of the CK-MB and LD1/LD in the Goldman test positive population is usually positive in AMI patients. The results of CK-MB positive with AMI improves 4 hours later, so the use of change of CK-MB. The contingency table does not show the amount of uncertainty resolved by combined CK-MB/%LD1.

CASE 3. CHEST PAIN AND A GOLDMINER (GRAPHICAL ORDINAL LOGIT DISPLAY) ESTIMATION

We here examine a cohort of 245 patients randomized into two groups. All patients presented to the emergency department with symptoms suggestive of acute myocardial infarct and were triaged in the usual manner using the chest pain criteria, ECG, and CK isoenzyme MB measured in serum at the time of presenting and at 3 and 12 hours later. Half the patients were tested for cardiac troponin T (cTnT) at times 0, 3, and 12 hours if they entered the randomized prospective trial. We are not concerned here with cTnT, but with the process of assessing the information used in decision making. Table 6 shows the frequencies and probabilities of chest pain and ECG findings

**Table 3   Goldman Algorithm
Results Versus Diagnosis of AMI,
as Frequency (Probability)**

Goldman	Diagnosis	
	Not AMI	**AMI**
Negative	33 (0.97)	1 (0.03)
Positive	30 (0.18)	137 (0.82)

Table 4 Means and SEM of CK-MB and LD1/LD Ratio for Diagnoses

Diagnosis	Test	Means	SEM
Not AMI	CK-MB 8 hrs	7.9 U/L	19.8
	LD1/LD	26.3%	2.2
AMI	CK-MB 8 hrs	93.5 U/L	10.0
	LD1/LD	43%	1.1

associated with AMI, angina, and not AMI. We examine the multivariable model more in another case study. The chest pain (CP) and ECG are scaled:

CP: 1, other; 2, atypical; 3, typical.
ECG: 1, other; 2, ST depression (STD) and LBBB; 3, ST elevation.

The fit of the model is significant with chi-square = 22.62 ($p = 4.8 \times 10^{-5}$). I do not show a table of the odds ratios in this example. The clinical features form classes that predict AMI, angina, and not AMI (NAMI).

The goodness of fit is tested by chi-square. One can compare the models for diagnoses using combinations as well as single variables by comparing the chi-squares for the single and joint variables. Table 7 compares the models using CP, ECG, CK-MB, and then replacing CK-MB with cTnT.

CASE 4. GOLDMINER (GRAPHICAL ORDINAL LOGIT DISPLAY): AN EASY-TO-USE METHOD FOR HANDLING ORDERED OUTCOMES—AN EXAMPLE USING OVARIAN CANCER REMISSION

The common approach to handling data with binary outcomes is logistic regression with a least squares fit of the data. This method gives unacceptable results when the distribution of the groups and residuals is not the same.

Magidson (Statistical Innovations, Inc., Belmont, MA) (Magidson, 1995, 1996) has developed a more general graphical model for analysis of a binary

Table 5 Frequency Table of CK-MB and LD1/LD for Diagnoses

Test result	Not AMI	AMI	
CK-MB			
Negative	23	25	48 (37.5%)
Positive	3	77	80 (62.5%)
LD1/LD			
Negative	18	10	28 (21.9%)
Positive	8	92	100 (78.1%)
	26 (20.3%)	102 (79.7%)	

Table 6   Frequency and Probability of Chest Pain (CP) and ECG Features in AMI, Angina, and Not AMI (NAMI) Diagnoses

CP/ECG	NAMI	Angina	AMI
1,1	8 (0.93)	0 (0.07)	0 (0)
2,1	21 (0.83)	4 (0.15)	0 (0.02)
1,2	4 (0.79)	1 (0.18)	0 (0.03)
3,1	31 (0.62)	15 (0.29)	6 (0.09)
2,2	1 (0.55)	0 (0.32)	1 (0.13)
3,2	4 (0.25)	6 (0.37)	2 (0.38)
2,3	0 (0.19)	0 (0.35)	2 (0.46)

response that is a nonlinear alternative to the standard approach. We use this model to illustrate the probabilistic representation of effects. The method displays the odds ratios for treatments versus responses. We apply the method to modeling a prediction of remission for ovarian cancer postoperatively using operative findings, stage, and CA_{125} half-life.

Study Population.   We examine a published data set. Data were analyzed from 55 women who were treated at Yale University, had an evaluable CA_{125} half-life ($t_{1/2}$), and were followed for disease recurrence for at least 3 years.

Universal regression to odds ratios.   We examine the associations between operative findings and CA_{125} to remission and nonremission or relapse using a universal regression model under an assumption of bivariate normality with estimation of generalized odds-ratios developed by Jay Magidson (Statistical Innovations, Inc., Belmont, MA)(Magidson, 1995, 1996). The universal regression model is a unified maximum likelihood method for assessing simultaneously both the statistical significance of treatment effects and the model fit when the response variable is ordered. It uses a parallel log-odds model based on adjacent odds to describe the data (Magidson, 1995, 1996).

The universal regression is carried out after scaling the continuous variables with intervals we determined as follows: half-life 0–5, 6–10, 11–15,

Table 7   Comparison of Chi-Square for GOLDminer Ordinal Class Models

Class	Chi-square	p
CP	8.22	0.0041
ECG	9.86	0.0017
CP/ECG	22.62	4.8×10^{-5}
CK-MB	9.21	0.0024
CP/ECG/CK-MB	34.31	1.7×10^{-7}
CP/ECG/cTnT	71.36	2.2×10^{-15}

16–20, >20. A cross-tabulation is constructed using the scaled variables as treatment versus the effect (full remission, short remission, or none), to obtain the frequency tabulation of treatment level versus remission, relapse, or nonremission. The data table is used for the universal regression. The cross-tabulation is of the number of events that are in each class (full remission, relapse, and nonremission) by predictor. The probabilities are regressed based on the level of the predictors being inversely related to the expected outcome. The results are presented in a GOLDminer plot. The goodness of fit is tested by the chi-square, shown at the top of the graph with the value of p. The XY view of the results should have a curvilinear response fitting the data points to the log(odds ratio)—in this case, low values with low log(odds ratio) versus high values with high log(odds ratio).

Results. The one-way analysis of variance (ANOVA1) of CA-125 half-life by operative findings is significant at $p = .01$ ($F[2,52] = 5.073$). The remission results of the outcome groups (means, standard error of mean (SEM), [N])(months) were as follows: Remission, 38.1, 2.8, [19]; Relapse, 18.8, 3.0, [16]; Nonremission, 0, [20]. Likewise, the means and SEM of HL (days) for the same outcome groups were as follows: Remission, 7.9, 2.8; Relapse, 17.4, 3.1; Nonremission, 17.4, 2.8. Relapse and failure to achieve remission were combined into one outcome class. The means and standard error of the means (SEM) of half-life versus remission or nonremission/relapse are effectively separated ($F = 7.42, p < 0.01$) as follows: Remission, 7.9, 2.8, [19]; Relapse/Nonremission, 17.4, 2.05, [36].

Table 8 is a cross-tabulation of the observed and expected outcome frequencies in remission (rem), short remission (short, <30 months) and nonremission (none) versus the scaled half-lives.

Table 9 is the expected odds that are calculated from the expected frequency and used to calculate expected odds ratio. The expected odds ratio is calculated from the odds by dividing the expected odds by the reference odds. The reference frequency is that for remission versus short or none. Dividing each cell by the frequency for remission results in the remis-

Table 8   Observed and Expected Frequencies of Remission, Relapse, and No Response by Half-Life

Half-life (range, days)	Observed frequency			Expected frequency		
	Rem	Short	None	Rem	Short	None
>20	0	4	5	0.40	1.68	6.92
16–20	0	0	2	0.25	0.55	1.20
11–15	4	8	8	5.64	6.63	7.73
6–10	12	3	5	9.93	6.21	3.85
<6	3	1	0	2.77	0.92	0.30

Table 9   Expected Odds and Expected Odds-Ratios for Remission, Relapse, and No Response by Half-Life

Half-life (range, days)	Exp. odds			Exp. odds ratios		
	Rem	Short	None	Rem	Short	None
>20	1	4.16	17.11	1	12.49	56.07
16–20	1	2.21	4.84	1	6.64	44.16
11–15	1	1.18	1.37	1	3.53	12.49
6–10	1	0.63	0.39	1	1.88	3.53
<6	1	0.33	0.11	1	1	1
HL-ref	1	0.33	0.11	1	1	1

sion column with all ones, and the other outcome odds shown. Dividing each cell by the reference expected odds gives the expected odds ratio. In this case the half-life days is set as the reference for expected odds and all the cells in that row convert to odds ratios of 1. Figure 2 is a plot of CA_{125} value versus information in bits (uncertainty resolved). Figure 3 is the Kaplan–Meier survival curves for CA_{125} half-life either less than or equal to, or greater than, 10 days.

Discussion.   We are able to regress the data so that half-life is associated with predicted odds for or against remission. In the example used there are three outcomes: remission, short remission, and none. If short remission and none were combined, then the analysis would be the same as a logistic

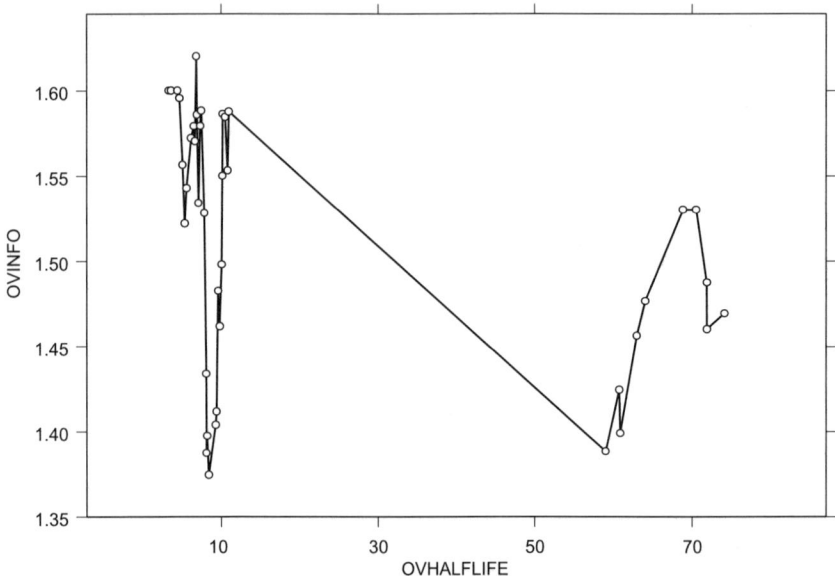

Figure 2 CA_{125} values plotted against the effective information (bits).

Kaplan-Meier Cumulative Survival Plot

Cumulative Proportion of Survival

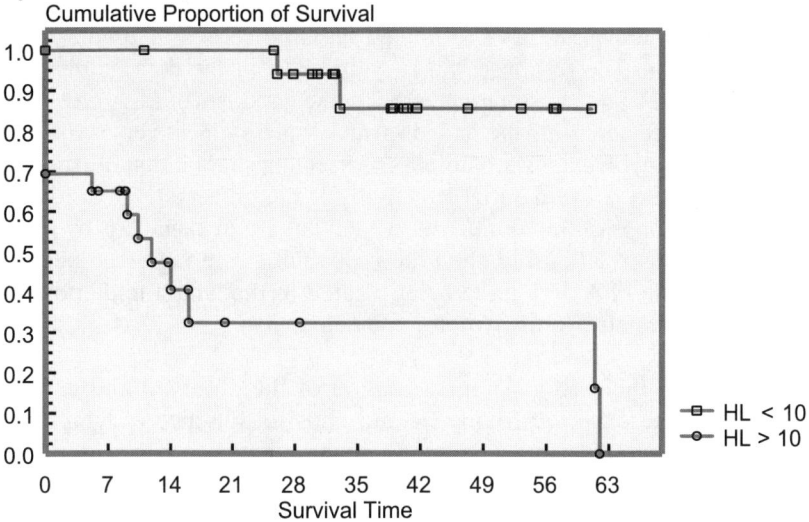

Figure 3   Kaplan-Meier survival curves for CA_{125} at 10-day cutoff.

regression. The logistic regression doesn't handle a situation with more than two outcomes. Using GOLDminer analysis with more than one predictor, such as operative findings and half-life, analogous to multiple linear regression, is omitted in this example.

CASE STUDY 5. GOLDMINER USING TWO PREDICTORS FOR PROSTATE CARCINOMA LYMPH-NODE EXTENSION

I describe the application of the GOLDminer and its output to the prediction of likelihood or not for lymph-node extension based on a combined probability model using PSA and pathological grade.

Objective.   Visualizing risk is important for studying outcomes. We use the new graphical ordinal regression (GOR) model to display odds ratios and illustrate the probabilistic representation of PSA and grade versus lymph-node positivity (Statistical Innovation, Belmont, MA). This would determine a minimum below which lymph-node extension is unlikely and a maximum above which lymph-node extension is likely, obviating the need for lymph node resection.

Data and methodology.   The data were provided and checked for accuracy by Dr. Gustave Davis from the Department of Pathology surgical registry. We classified the data using these variables by mapping the results into a self-classifying matrix as described by Rypka (1992) and by Rudolph et al. (1988). The GOR is carried out after scaling the PSA and grade, respectively: <5, 5–13.9, 14–21.9, 22–35.9, 36–59, >59; <5, 5–6, 7, >7. GOR is done using univariate and combined variable classes to predict lymph node extension. The response is a curvilinear fit of the data points to the log(odds ratios) with chi-square measuring the goodness of fit. A cross-tabulation is constructed using the scaled variables as treatment versus the effect (lymph-node involvement), to obtain the frequency tabulation of treatment level versus effect. The data table is used for the universal regression. The cross-tabulation is of the number of events that are in each class by predictor. If there is a relationship, then the probabilities are regressed based on the level of the PSA and grade being related to the lymph-node positivity and inversely related to the lymph-node negativity.

Results. Table 10 is a representation of the observed and expected counts, and the expected frequency and odds for absence of lymph-node involvement based on the PSA/grade classes shown. Absence of lymph-node involvement is only predictable at PSA level below 5 ng/mL and grade less than 5.

Table 11 is a representation of the observed and expected counts, and the expected frequency and odds for lymph-node involvement based on the PSA/grade classes shown. Lymph-node extension is expected at PSA level exceeding 36 and grade above 7. Table 12 is a nongraphical view of GOLD-miner, shown in Figure 4. The goodness-of-fit is tested by chi-square. A curvilinear response fits the data points to the log(odds ratio)—in this case, low values with low log(odds ratio) versus high values with high log(odds ratio). The ordinal regression gives the best fit of the data. The chi-square is 41.5 for the fit, significant at $p = 1.2 \times 10^{-10}$.

Table 10   Frequencies for PSA and Grade Versus Negative Lymph-Node Status

PSA/Grade	Observed counts	Expected counts	Expected frequency	Expected odds
>36, >7	1	0.40	0.20	0.80
<22, >7	1	0.49	0.24	0.83
>36, 7	1	2.10	0.42	0.95
>59, 5–6	2	3.31	0.55	1.03
>36, 5–6	2	4.06	0.68	1.13
<22, 7	3	2.93	0.73	1.18
<36, 5–6	12	10.16	0.78	1.23
<14, 7	6	6.59	0.82	1.28
<22, 5–6	15	15.51	0.91	1.46
<14, 5–6	28	28.88	0.93	1.52
<22, <5	9	8.63	0.96	1.66
<14, < 5	37	36.79	0.97	1.73

Table 11   Frequencies for PSA and Grade Versus Positive Lymph-Node Status

PSA/Grade	Observed counts	Expected counts	Expected frequency	Expected odds
<36, >7	1	1.60	0.80	3.22
<22, >7	1	1.51	0.76	2.57
>36, 7	4	2.90	0.58	1.31
>59, 5–6	4	2.69	0.45	0.84
>36, 5–6	4	1.94	0.32	0.54
<22, 7	1	1.07	0.27	0.43
<36, 5–6	1	2.84	0.22	0.34
<14, 7	2	1.41	0.18	0.27
<22, 5–6	2	1.49	0.09	0.44
<14, 5–6	3	2.12	0.07	0.11
<22, <5	0	0.37	0.04	0.07
<14, <5	1	1.21	0.03	0.06

Conclusions.   The GOR model extends classification of data into the realm of risk and outcomes.

CASE STUDY 6. MALNUTRITION CLINICAL PATHWAY

Linda Brugler, RD, and Marie DiPrinzio, RN, MBA, of St. Francis Hospital, Wilmington, DE, have designed a malnutrition clinical pathway. Data was collected for comparable periods in 1996 and 1997, before and after initiating the pathway. Scaling was done of length of hospital stay (LOS), intensive

Table 12   Odds Ratios for PSA and Grade Versus Lymph-Node Extension

	Lymph-node involvement			
	Negative		Positive	
PSA/Grade	Observed counts	Odds ratio	Observed counts	Odds ratio
<36, 7	1	0.56	1	19.89
<22, >7	1	0.59	1	15.90
>36, 7	1	0.67	4	8.12
>59, 5–6	2	0.73	4	5.19
>36, 5–6	2	0.80	4	3.32
<22, 7	3	0.83	1	2.65
<36, 5–6	12	0.87	1	2.12
<14, 7	6	0.90	2	0.90
<22, 5–6	15	1.03	2	0.87
<14, 5–6	28	1.07	3	0.69
<22,	9	1.17	0	0.44
<14, <5	37	1.22	1	0.35

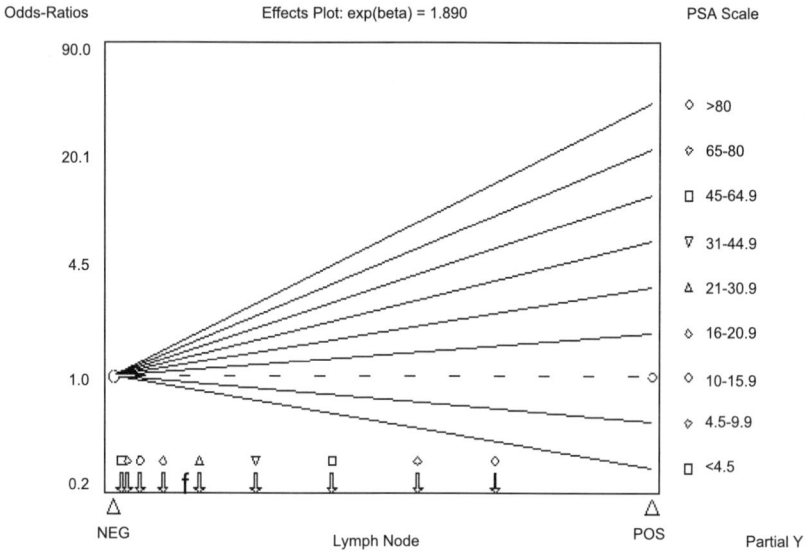

Figure 4 GOLDminer plot of PSA versus lymph-node extension.

care days, admitting serum albumin, number of dietitian visits, and days of intervention. A convenient rule was as follows: none, 9; 1–5, 1; 6–10, 2; 11–15, 3; 16–20, 4; >20, 5. Variables used to predict outcomes, such as LOS, discharge disposition, and complications, were albumin, functionality, and use of specialized nutrition support (enteral or parenteral). The study required the data sets to be examined and normalized for severity of illness using scaled values of serum albumin (Figure 5). These were: >2.7 g/dl, 2.3–2.7 g/dl, and <2.3 g/dl.

Results. The data from the periods compared show significant relations among albumin level, LOS, complications, and functional status. The levels of albumin, functional status (ability to function independently), and complications were scaled and used in a risk model based on an additive risk score. The relationship between risk and the factors—albumin, functional status, and complication—is constructed in a multivariable GOLDminer plot displayed in Figure 6.

The effect of severity of illness as it relates to albumin level on LOS and complications needs to be accounted for in order to measure the effectiveness of the metabolic treatment program. Albumin level of the high-risk-for-malnutrition patient is strongly associated with LOS, complications, functional status at discharge, type of nutrition intervention required, and number of dietitian interventions needed. Figure 7 is a plot of interventions by a nutritionist versus LOS.

Comparison of ANOVA Cell Means
F = 10.88721, p = .0001

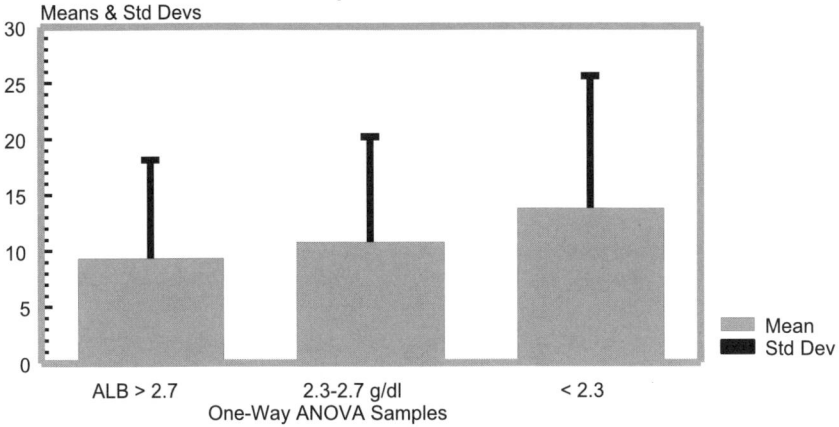

Figure 5 Relationship of scaled albumin values to LOS.

The important point that we learned from the study is that while number of interventions tracks LOS, timely and frequent intervention reduces LOS compared with an unmanaged cohort. All patients in the study received case-mix weighting. An analysis of the means of the retrospective and prospective study groups for variables of interest is similar ($p = 0.06$). We carried out cross-tabulations to examine the frequency of subgroups in

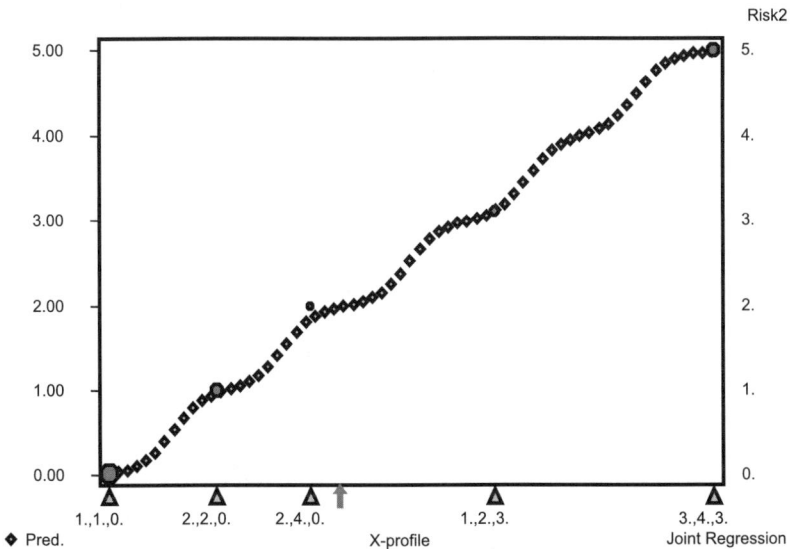

Figure 6 GOLDminer multivariable regression of factors versus risk.

Least Squares Means

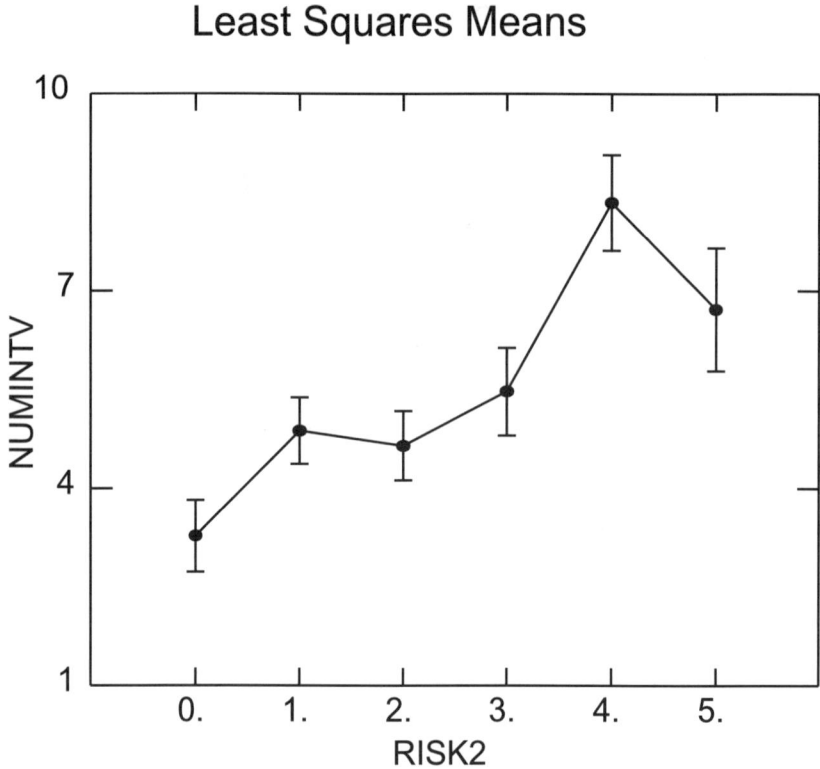

Figure 7   Relationship between risk and nutritionist interventions.

the retrospective versus prospective study for albumin based on the described values >2.7 g/dl, 2.3–2.7 g/dl, and <2.3 g/dl, and for subgroups of two case-mix classes based on a cutoff of 1.5 weight. The frequencies of the classes formed by combining case-mix and albumin intervals into six classes were (Table 13): "11," 127, 110; "12," 50, 53; "13," 47, 53; "21," 45, 31; "22," 20, 19; "23," 27, 34. The LOS in case-mix >1.5 and albumin <2.3 (23), for the retrospective versus prospective study is 16 and 22.4 days. What is most striking is that "11," "12," and "13" are at one level, "21" and "22" another, and "23" a third level of LOS, and the albumin has an effect over the case-mix in separating cases based on LOS (and resource use).

The classes "12," "13," and "23" were of interest in describing differences between studies. These had a 1.9%, 2.8%, and 2.8% greater frequency in the prospective set, which could be applied to 300 patients (6.5%). If the severity is adjusted to the same frequency for prospective as retrospective, there would be 23 patients and at 8.8, 10.3, and 20 days LOS for 12, 13, and 23, a total of 305 days. The total average LOS is 10 days, which results in 30 clinical events at a cost of $14,000 an event, or an annual cost saving of $1,008,000. This example illustrates how use of cross-table analysis allows us

Table 13 Frequencies of Classes in Matched Time Periods

Class	Case-mix	Albumin	Study 1 frequency	Study 2 frequency
"11"	<1.5	>2.7	127	110
"12"	<1.5	2.3–2.7	50	53
"13"	<1.5	<2.3	47	53
"21"	≥1.5	>2.7	45	31
"22"	≥.5	2.3–2.7	20	19
"23"	≥1.5	<2.3	27	34

to compare two study groups after adjusting for comparable severity of illness based on frequency of patients within subgroups of high-risk, low albumin concentrations.

CONCLUSIONS

The laboratory has sufficient reason to be engaged in outcome research, which is allied with the discipline of clinical epidemiology. The emergence of a laboratory-based epidemiology is compelling because laboratory information makes a large contribution to the information used for making clinical decisions. A laboratory-based epidemiology is grounded on extending our quality activities beyond traditional quality control of data to quality control of the information product.

I have attempted to outline the methods that can be used without great difficulty to carry out outcome studies using laboratory data. The framework for many questions of the nature of hypothesis testing is grounded in construction of the 2-by-2 contingency table. The main problem with such an approach is that it does not lead to alternative hypotheses if the "null hypothesis" is rejected. The use of n-by-n contingency tables becomes useful for examining relationships with more than two variables. I also describe the formation of "truth tables," which are lists of classes described by their key defining features and the formal method for feature extraction. The main purpose of this is that all potential hypotheses that can be identified are represented by the pattern classes. I call attention to the observation by Mayzlin and Bernstein (unpublished) that a nonlinear training algorithm, the artificial neural network by backpropagation, can be trained using a classification method for preprocessing the data. The most commonly used methods for health services research are linear regression based on OLS or a logistic regression. The first uses R^2 comparing variance within each cell versus variance of population, as a measure of fit. The second measures dichotomous outcomes and uses the c-statistic as a measure of fit. Classic statistical assumptions may be violated in using these methods. I present case studies and examples using a new method, universal regression, introduced by Jay Magidson at Statistical Innovations (Belmont, MA) and available in software form as GOLDminer from SPSS.

REFERENCES

Draper N, Smith H. *Applied Regression Analysis*, second edition. Wiley, New York, 1981.

Galen RS, Gambino SR. *Beyond Normality: The Predictive Value and Efficiency of Medical Diagnosis*. John Wiley & Sons, New York, 1975.

Goldman L, Weinberg M, et al. A computer derived protocol to aid in the diagnosis of emergency room patients with acute chest pain. *N. Engl. J. Med.* 1982;307:588–596.

Goldman L, Cook EF, Brand DA, et al. A computer protocol to predict myocardial infarction in emergency department patients with chest pain. *N. Engl. J. Med.* 1988;318:797–803.

Haberman SJ. Computation of maximum likelihood estimates in association models. *J. Am. Stat. Assoc.* 1995;90:1438–1446.

Hayes WL. *Statistics*, third edition. Holt, Rhinehart and Winston, New York, 1981.

Iezzone LI. Chapters 1-4. In Iezzone LI, ed., *Risk Adjustment for Measuring Healthcare Outcomes*, second edition. Health Administration Press, Chicago, 1997.

Jekel JF, Elmore JG, Katz DL. Understanding and reducing errors in clinical medicine. In *Epidemiology, Biostatistics, and Preventive Medicine,* pp. 87–97. W. B. Saunders, Philadelphia, 1996a.

Jekel JF, Elmore JG, Katz DL. Bivariate analysis. In *Epidemiology, Biostatistics, and Preventive Medicine,* pp. 139–158. W. B. Saunders, Philadelphia, 1996b.

Kooperberg C, Bose S, Stone CJ. Polychotomous regression. *J. Am. Stat. Assoc.* 1997;92:117–127.

Krieg AF, Gambino SR, Galen RS. Why clinical laboratory tests are performed and their validity. In Lundberg GD (ed.), *Using the Clinical Laboratory in Medical Decision-Making*, pp. 229–233. American Society for Clinical Pathology Press, Chicago, 1983.

Littenberg B, Moses LE. Estimating diagnostic accuracy from multiple conflicting reports: A new meta-analytic method. *Med. Decision Making* 1993;13:313–321.

Magidson J. Introducing a new graphical model for the analysis of an ordered categorical response—Part I. *J. Targeting Measure. Anal. Market.* 1995;4(2): 133–148.

Magidson J. Maximum likelihood assessment of clinical trials based on an ordered categorical response. *Drug Inform. J.* 1996;30(1):143–170.

Martin HF, Gudzinowicz BJ, Fanger H. *Normal Values in Clinical Chemistry: A Guide to Statistical Analysis of Laboratory Data*, Marcel Dekker, New York, 1975.

Mozes B, Easterling MJ, Sheiner LB, Melmon KL, et al. Case-mix adjustment using objective measures of severity: The case for laboratory data. *Health Serv. Res.* 1994; 28:689–711.

Qu Y, Hagdu A. A model for evaluating sensitivity and specificity for correlated diagnostic tests in efficacy studies with an imperfect reference. *J. Am. Stat. Assoc.* 1998;93:920–928

Rudolph RA, Bernstein LH, Babb J. Information induction for the diagnosis of myocardial infarction. *Clin. Chem.* 1988;34: 2031–2038.

Rypka EW. Methods to evaluate and develop the decision process in the selection of tests. In McPherson RA, Nakamura RM (eds.), *Clinics in Laboratory Medicine. Laboratory Immunology. II. Strategies for Clinical Laboratory Management,* vol. 12, pp. 351–386. W. B. Saunders, Philadelphia, 1992.

Selterman D, Louis TA. Contingency tables in medical studies. In Bailar JC III, Mosteller F (eds.), *Medical Uses of Statistics,* second edition. New England Journal of Medicine Books, Boston, 1992.

Shaw-Stiffel TA, Zarny LA, Pleban WE, Rosman DD, Rudolph RA, Bernstein LH. Effect of nutritional status and other factors on length of stay following major GI surgery. *Nutrition* 1993;9:1–6.

Speicher CE, Smith JW. *Choosing Effective Laboratory Tests,* pp. 47–59. W. B. Saunders, Philadelphia, 1983.

APPENDIX

Clustering: Grouping of similar objects. Formal, planned, purposeful, or scientific classification. It is necessary in taxonomy for the same objects to have the same classification. A common way to classify is by using geometric distance clustering. The method measures similarity by measuring the distance between objects and constructs a classification so that the distances between related objects within the clusters is small. Errors are greatest in classifying when the distance between objects within clusters is large compared with distances between clusters.

Decision level: The decision level of a test is the value for the variable that best relieves uncertainty in the data set. At the maximum entropy decision level of a variable, the variable used in combination with other variables can be used to form a binary pattern to classify the data with the least number of classification errors.

Effective information: This is also known as Kullback entropy. It is the difference in entropy between the maximum entropy and the data entropy, obtained by subtracting the entropy in the data set, at given decision points, from the entropy of the randomized data in which associations are destroyed.

Group-based reference: When more than one variable is available, the data may contain enough information to differentiate between disease and nondisease by measuring the uncertainty, or missing information in the data set. The data form complementary disease and healthy-reference subsets defining the population by the observational attributes. The healthy-reference subset, like the statistical null set, contains no information and it reflects maximum uncertainty. The disease subset contains the information needed to relieve uncertainty.

Entropy and information theory. Entropy is the quantitative measure of information in a message transmission. The information of the message set is the entropy, H:

$$H = P_1 \log_2(1/P_1) + P_2 \log_2(1/P) + \cdots + P_n \log_2(1/P_n)$$

Port Royal classes. Formal methods for classification of diseases require describing terms by attributes that would verify the uniqueness of the term(s). Applying a formal method to a large data base would allow for unique definition of classes based on objective observations.

Rypka's S-clustering. Consider four essential maneuvers: (1) scaling, (2) calculation of S-values, (3) horizontal rearrangement of features, and (4) vertical rearrangement of elements (patients). This creates a primary classification that accurately maps to the truth table.

Section III

Practical Applications

Chapter 9

Laboratory Tests for Case-Finding and Screening for Disease in the Ambulatory Setting

M. D. Silverstein

Advances in medical knowledge; development of new tests, drugs, devices, and procedures; and the aging of the U.S. population have all contributed to the increase in health care cost in recent years. Changes in the organization and financing of health care have shifted some health care services from the hospital to ambulatory setting, have increased interest in primary care and prevention, and have altered the financial incentives for ordering laboratory tests (Relman, 1988; Eisenberg et al., 1987). Guidelines, clinical pathways, and procedures have been implemented to reduce variations in testing, control cost, and improve outcomes. It is therefore timely to focus on laboratory tests in the ambulatory setting. This chapter provides a clinician's perspective on the role of laboratory tests for case-finding in the ambulatory setting.

Clinical laboratories include hospital-based laboratories, freestanding laboratories, and laboratories located in physicians' offices. Laboratories receive specimens from hospital patients in multiple settings (inpatient service, intensive care units, operative suite, and the ambulatory clinic), as well as specimens from patients in nursing homes or physicians' offices. The laboratorian is more often likely to focus on the laboratory, the type of laboratory tests (clinical, chemistry, microbiology, etc.), or specific laboratory tests. The laboratorian is often consulted to assist in the interpretation of tests ordered for diagnostic evaluation of hospitalized patients with complex conditions or serious illness and advice on additional testing. The laboratorian should be equally well prepared to advise clinicians and administrators on the role of laboratory tests for case-finding and screening in the ambulatory setting.

There are many indications for ordering laboratory tests. Laboratory tests are obtained in the evaluation of patients with known or suspected disease (diagnosis), for following severity of disease or response to therapy(monitoring), to predict the future course of disease (prognosis), or to identify unsuspected disease (case-finding). In the hospital setting, most tests are obtained for diagnostic evaluation and monitoring. In the ambulatory setting of the periodic health examination, the majority of laboratory tests are ordered for case-finding (Boland, 1996). Thus laboratorians should be familiar with the issues of case-finding in the ambulatory setting and understand the potential impact of changes in health care on test ordering and the demand for laboratory tests. Laboratorians should be able to work with clinicians and other providers to maximize efficient and appropriate use of laboratory services for ambulatory patients whose care occurs in the managed-care setting.

DEFINITIONS

Laboratorians, clinicians, managers, and health services researchers may use the same terms in different contexts and with different meanings. It is therefore useful to define four terms that are used to describe the role of laboratory tests and other health services in the ambulatory setting (Silverstein, 1989). These definitions were originally developed by the Canadian Task Force on the Periodic Health Examination (CTPHE, 1979) (Table 1).

Screening refers to the use of laboratory tests and other procedures in the unselected general population to identify persons with an increased risk of death, disease, or disability due to disease. The persons identified to have an increased risk are advised to consult their physician or another provider for further follow-up. Persons who are tested in a screening program may not have a primary care physician or an established relationship with a health-care provider. Accordingly, those responsible for the screening program have an ethical obligation to those screened to assure that persons identified with a high-risk condition have access to follow-up care for further evaluation and treatment.

Case-finding refers to the use of laboratory tests (and other procedures) by a physician or other health-care provider for a patient to detect an unsuspected condition that is unrelated to the problem for which the patient is consulting a health-care professional. The health-care provider who ordered the test is responsible for further evaluation or referral of the patient to other health-care professionals for further evaluation and treatment. The terms "screening" and "case-finding" are often confused, and "screening" is sometimes used to describe case-finding in the ambulatory setting. Testing newborn babies for sickle-cell disease is screening; ordering a lipid profile as part of periodic health exam is case-finding.

Screening generally refers to testing the general population. An important distinction is the use of laboratory tests for *selected* populations.

Table 1   Definitions

Term	Definition
Screening	The use of procedures in unselected populations to classify the populations into two groups: those with a high probability of being affected by fatal or disabling condition and a group with a low probability.
Case-finding	Detection of disease by means of tests or procedures undertaken by health workers on patients who are consulting a health worker for unrelated symptoms or unrelated reasons.
Efficacy	Attribute of an intervention or maneuver that results in more good than harm to those who accept and comply with the intervention and subsequent treatment.
Effectiveness	Attribute of an intervention or maneuver that results in more good than harm to those to whom it is offered.

Laboratorians should understand the underlying population that is being screened because the test characteristics, prevalence of disease, and test performance may vary in different populations. The use of cholesterol and other laboratory tests in the general population sample for the U.S. National Health and Nutrition Examination Survey (NHANES) is an excellent example of screening. Cholesterol testing at a shopping mall or in a local "health fair" is an example of screening a selected population. The prevalence of hyperlipidemia (and previously undiagnosed hyperlipidemia), the sensitivity and specificity of the cholesterol tests, and predictive value of cholesterol screening in these selected populations will be different in those who visit shopping malls and agree to be tested and in those self-selected attendees of "health fairs" than in the general population.

Efficacy and *effectiveness* are useful concepts, and laboratorians and clinicians should be aware of the distinction in these terms and, more importantly, consider the type of study and nature of the evidence for the use of laboratory tests for screening and case-finding. Efficacy describes the performance of a test under ideal conditions and in clinical trials. In contrast, effectiveness describes the performance of the laboratory tests under usual conditions. While tests must be efficacious in order to be effective in the ambulatory setting, tests that are efficacious for diagnoses in the hospital setting may be less effective for case-finding or may not be effective for case-finding in the ambulatory setting.

The populations included in efficacy and effectiveness definitions differ. The more limited the inclusion and exclusion criteria are in clinical trials and in other studies of new tests, drugs, and devices, the more likely it is that they will result in a different spectrum of disease in the patients studied than in the patients seen in the usual practice. In clinical trials, patients with the disease often have more severe disease, and patients without the disease may be healthier or less likely to have other comorbid conditions (Ranso-hoff and Feinstein, 1978).

The test characteristics reported in efficacy studies may not reflect their performance in patients in the ambulatory setting. This means that tests may have lower sensitivity and specificity when applied in the ambulatory set-ting. Since the proportion of persons with disease is usually higher in study populations than the prevalence of the disease in the general population of ambulatory patients, the predictive value positive and predictive value nega-tive of laboratory tests will be lower when ordered for case-finding.

Efficacy studies are more likely to be reported in the laboratory medi-cine journals, and effectiveness studies are more likely to be reported in clinical journals. Effectiveness of commonly available laboratory tests for case-finding has not been extensively investigated. Thus, laboratorians may not be aware of the existing effectiveness literature and should hesitate to make inferences about the effectiveness of laboratory tests for case-finding based on studies of the efficacy of laboratory tests for diagnostic evaluation of patients with a different spectrum of disease.

CRITERIA FOR SCREENING AND CASE-FINDING

The World Health Organization formalized basic criteria for screening, which have been modified and restated in different ways over the years but have withstood the test of time (Wilson and Junger, 1968). These criteria also apply to the use of laboratory tests for case-finding in the ambulatory setting. A laboratory test that meets these criteria in the ambulatory setting can be recommended for case-finding, and a laboratory test that meets these criteria for the general population can be recommended for screening the general population (Table 2). Essentially, the criteria for screening and case-finding require that conditions be significant and amenable to early detection, that acceptable tests and treatments are available, and that treatment of screened detected disease should be effective and cost-effective. Most importantly, treatment of conditions detected by screening or case-finding should yield better results than treatment when the condition would otherwise become symptomatic. This is a key criterion, and most often evidence to fulfill this criterion is lacking when then the other criteria are met.

Unfortunately, there have been relatively few studies of the effective-ness of laboratory tests for case-finding. Randomized clinical trials of mul-tiphasic screening were conducted more than two decades ago and failed to find evidence of the effectiveness of laboratory tests as part of multiphasic screening (Friedman et al., 1986). Nevertheless, laboratory tests continue to be obtained in the ambulatory setting for case-finding. Many common con-ditions can be detected by these low-risk and low-cost laboratory tests. Patients want laboratory tests and have learned to expect to have laboratory tests included as part of their annual physical exam or periodic health examination. Patients and their physicians are reassured by negative or

Table 2   Criteria for Screening

Criteria	Description
Significant condition	The condition must have a significant effect on the quality or quantity of life.
Detectable period	The condition must have an asymptomatic period during which detection and treatment significantly reduce morbidity and mortality.
Acceptable tests	Tests acceptable to patients must be available at reasonable cost to detect the condition in the asymptomatic phase.
Acceptable treatment	Acceptable methods of treatment must be available.
Effectiveness	Treatment in the asymptomatic phase must yield a therapeutic result superior to that obtained by delaying treatment until symptoms appear.
Cost-effectiveness	Incidence of the condition must be sufficient to justify the cost of screening.

normal test results. Physicians and other providers frequently identify suspected disease as a result of ordering tests, and these new diagnoses reinforce clinicians' perceptions of the value of laboratory tests for case-finding in the ambulatory setting.

CONCEPTUAL FRAMEWORK FOR EVALUATING LABORATORY TESTS

A conceptual framework has been developed to assist in the evaluation of laboratory tests that are still frequently ordered in the ambulatory setting (Silverstein and Boland, 1994). The conceptual framework can be used to develop measures of the value of laboratory tests that may not meet all the criteria for screening and case-finding. This framework can be used in the evaluation of the commonly ordered tests that were shown not to reduce mortality or disability in randomized controlled trials (Olsen et al., 1976; Friedman et al., 1986) and therefore do not meet the criteria for screening. Such a conceptual framework is helpful in providing measures of the yield of laboratory tests for case-finding that can be used to inform decisions about test ordering (Table 2). The framework addresses the performance characteristics of the test in detecting disease, in establishing new diagnoses, in changing patient management, and in changing patient outcomes. The framework considers efficacy and, more importantly, the effectiveness of laboratory tests in the usual patient care setting. The framework asks four questions, and suggests useful measures for the yield of testing.

- What are the performance characteristics of the test?
- What is the effectiveness of the test in establishing new diagnoses?

- What is the impact of the laboratory test in changing patient management?
- What is the impact of the test on patient outcomes?

PREOPERATIVE LABORATORY TESTS

Patients with medical conditions for which surgery is indicated generally have extensive diagnostic evaluation, including laboratory tests, for diagnosis and monitoring their medical condition prior to surgery. In this context, laboratory tests have obvious value in patient management. Laboratory tests are simple, safe, and effective in detecting disease in ambulatory patients prior to surgery or for inpatient evaluation when decisions about surgery are being made. It is a natural extension of the indications for laboratory tests to obtain a battery or panel of tests for patients scheduled for surgery in order to identify patients with an increased risk of preventable postoperative complications. Preoperative laboratory tests are case-finding tests for the outcome of a surgical complication. Thus, lessons learned in the evaluation of the effectiveness of preoperative laboratory tests in reducing postoperative complications may be useful in evaluating the effectiveness of routine laboratory tests for case-finding for other conditions in the ambulatory setting.

Preoperative laboratory testing prior to surgery was widely adopted with a goal to reduce the risk of postoperative complications. Indeed once protocols became established it was difficult to conduct studies to evaluate the effectiveness of preoperative laboratory tests, partly based on concerns about litigation and a desire to obtain the best possible patient outcomes. It is difficult to find randomized controlled trials of preoperative tests that randomly allocated patients to a "no test" group. Nevertheless, a growing number of observational studies of preoperative laboratory tests have provided a new perspective on routine preoperative laboratory tests. The studies indicate that there is a high use but a low yield of preoperative tests. Abnormal test results are often not noted in the medical record, and often there is no evidence that the management of the patient changed in response to the abnormal laboratory test. Finally, abnormal laboratory tests are actually poor predictors of postoperative complications. A few selected studies will be described that support these findings. A study of over 1000 patients who had preoperative tests prior to elective cholecystectomy found that 5% of the 5003 routine tests were abnormal, and only 2% were considered potentially important. Management was changed for 1.6% of patients, and only 0.4% could have benefited from the test (Turnbull and Buck, 1987). In another study of 2000 elective surgical patients, only 0.5% of 126 routine tests were abnormal and only 0.2% were judged to indicate a surgically important result (Kaplan et al., 1985). Two studies from the Mayo Clinic show how the results have been used to change test ordering practices. A Mayo Clinic study of 3782 healthy adults, ASA class 1, who had routine preoperative testing found 4.2% with at least one abnormal result. Eighteen percent of the abnormalities could have been predicted from medical history or physical examination. Twenty-nine percent of the persons with abnormalities had further testing, and in only 0.26% of cases was management changed. No adverse effects were related to preoperative test results (Narr et al., 1991). The Mayo Clinic preoperative test guidelines were changed to eliminate routine tests in healthy adults of ages less than 40, to obtain only creatinine and glucose in healthy adults of ages 40 to 60, and to obtain creatinine, glucose, electrocardiogram, and chest radiograph in adults of age 60 or older. Patients who are taking a diuretic or who received a bowel preparation have a serum potassium; patients with history of cardiac or pulmonary disease have a chest radiograph; and smokers older than age 40 have spirometry (Silverstein and Boland, 1994). After the Mayo Clinic preoperative laboratory testing guidelines were implemented, a follow-up study was performed to evaluate the outcomes of patients who had no routine preoperative laboratory testing following a preoperative evaluation that consisted of a medical history and physical examination. A random sample of 1044 adults who underwent surgical or diagnostic procedures with anesthesia and no routine laboratory tests revealed no deaths or perioperative mortality. Intraoperative tests and postoperative tests were obtained as indicated, and none of these tests changed management. Thus, patients assessed by history and physical examination can safely undergo anesthesia and surgery with testing only as indicated intraoperatively and postoperatively (Narr et al., 1997). Implementation of guidelines for laboratory testing preoperatively as part of a continuous quality improvement process can reduce utilization, increase the appropriateness of test ordering, and result in substantial savings in health-care costs (Nardella et al., 1995).

LABORATORY TESTS FOR CASE-FINDING IN THE AMBULATORY SETTING

The laboratory tests that are frequently obtained in the ambulatory setting for case-finding include the complete blood count, chemistry panel, lipid panel, thyroid hormone test, and urinalysis. These tests can be used to detect abnormal function resulting from disease, and for some conditions, they are sufficient to confirm a diagnosis. These tests are certainly useful to monitor severity of disease or to monitor therapy.

The use of these laboratory tests for case-finding in the ambulatory setting must be evaluated in the context of the criteria for screening. This shifts the focus to prevalent, morbid, disabling conditions that have an asymptomatic period in the ambulatory patient. A complete blood count can detect anemia most often due to iron or folate deficiency or to blood loss. A chemistry panel could identify diabetes mellitus, hyperuricemia, hyperparathyroidism, or evidence of liver, bone, or kidney disease. Lipid profiles are diagnostic tests for the hyperlipidemias. Urinalysis could identify urinary tract infection, diabetes mellitus, kidney disease, or genitourinary tract malignancy (Ruttiman and Clemencon, 1994). Except for hyperlipidemia and diabetes, the prevalence of these conditions is very low in ambulatory adults.

The yield of laboratory tests for case-finding cannot be higher than the prevalence of disease in the population tested. Although these conditions can be detected, there is insufficient evidence that treatment of these conditions detected by laboratory tests for case-finding (screen detected disease) is superior to treatment initiated when the patient's condition would otherwise become symptomatic. Accordingly, the use of these laboratory tests for case-finding for these conditions is generally not currently recommended because these tests fail to meet the WHO criteria for screening and case-finding.

There are only a few studies of laboratory tests for case-finding in the ambulatory setting. The best known study is the Kaiser-Permanente study of multiphasic testing. This was a randomized controlled trial of the periodic health checkup. In this study, 5156 randomly selected health plan members ages 35 to 54 were advised to have annual multiphasic screening, including automated multichannel laboratory tests. The control group of 5557 health plan members received usual care. After 16 years of follow-up there were no differences in total mortality or disability attributed to any laboratory test component of the multiphasic checkup. There was a 30% reduction in predefined postponable causes of death that was largely due to reduction in deaths due to hypertension and colorectal cancer (Friedman et al., 1986). Another study of multiphasic testing in 574 families found no differences in health status or morbidity but an increase in hospital utilization in the screened subjects (Olsen et al., 1976). These studies are important because they were randomized controlled trials and took place in the usual ambulatory care setting. These were effectiveness studies. The large number of patients enrolled in the studies and long-term follow-up in the Kaiser-Permanente study of the multiphasic checkup are strong evidence against the routine ordering of laboratory tests for case-finding in ambulatory adults.

Recent studies of laboratory tests for case-finding from a university general internal medicine clinic in Basel, Switzerland, and from general internal medicine practices at the Mayo Clinic in Rochester, Minnesota, have reported diagnostic yield and therapeutic yield of laboratory tests for case-finding (Table 3). Ruttiman and colleagues from Basel, Switzerland, prospectively studied 493 patients who had a 23-item biochemistry panel that included lipids. The diagnostic yield of the biochemistry/lipid panel was 5.1% and the therapeutic yield was 4%. Two-thirds of new diagnoses were hyperlipidemia. The study found that all clinically important abnormalities were detected by three tests: cholesterol, glucose, and alanine aminotransferase (Ruttiman et al., 1993) (Table 4). A study of the complete blood count in 595 adults from the same clinic found a diagnostic yield of 0.8% and a therapeutic yield of 0.3% (Ruttiman et al., 1992). The mean age of patients in these two studies was approximately 40 years. The low prevalence of

Table 3   Framework for Evaluating Laboratory Tests for Case-Finding

Criteria	Description	Measures
Test performance	Does the test detect disease?	Sensitivity, specificity, positive and negative predictive value.
Diagnosis	Is the test effective in establishing new diagnoses when ordered for case-finding in the usual patient care setting?	Sensitivity, specificity, positive and negative predictive value. *Diagnostic yield*: proportion of persons for whom the test is ordered for case-finding result in a new diagnosis.
Management	Does the laboratory test ordered for case-finding in the usual patient care setting result in a change in patient management?	*Therapeutic yield:* proportion of persons for whom the test is ordered for case-finding result in a new diagnosis associated with a change in management.
Patient outcome	Does the laboratory test ordered for case-finding in the usual patient care setting result in changes in management that change patient outcome?	Mortality, life expectancy, function, disability, quality-adjusted life years (QALYs), cost.

disease in this relatively young group of patients, and perhaps, different diagnostic thresholds for initiating treatment of hyperlipidemia, may explain, in part, the low diagnostic and therapeutic yield.

Similar results were found in two studies from the Mayo Clinic. In the first study, the records of 100 patients who had a comprehensive general medical examination and routine tests were reviewed. The complete blood count, a 12-item chemistry panel, a thyroid hormone test (either a sensitive thyroid-stimulating hormone [sTSH] or a serum thyroxine [T_4]), a lipid panel, and a urinalysis ordered for case-finding were evaluated. The lipid profile had the highest diagnostic yield (12.3%) and therapeutic yield (9.2%). The other tests had a diagnostic yield of 1–3% and a therapeutic yield of 1–2%. Of interest was that the review of systems had a diagnostic yield of 11% and a therapeutic yield of 7%, and the physical examination had a diagnostic yield of 9% and a therapeutic yield of 5%; both maneuvers had a higher yield than the laboratory tests, except for lipids (Boland et al., 1995). While the conditions detected by review of systems and physical examination differ from those detected by laboratory tests ordered for case-finding, it is useful to consider these different maneuvers, especially in

Table 4 Laboratory Tests for Case-Finding in the Ambulatory Setting

Study, Year	Setting	Patients	Test	Case-finding tests	Diagnostic yield,* no. (%)	Therapeutic yield,* no. (%)	Comment
Ruttimann et al., 1992	Basel, Switzerland, University General Internal Medicine Clinic	595, Age 40 ± 16, 38% female	CBC (4 items)	595	5 (1.5)	3 (0.9)	Iron deficiency anemia
Ruttimann et al., 1993	Basel, Switzerland, University General Internal Medicine Clinic	493, Age 41 ± 15, 43% female	Biochemistry & lipid panel (23 items)	493	48 (9.7)	25 (5.1)	All clinically important diagnoses resulted from lipids cholesterol, glucose, and ALT**
Boland et al., 1995	Rochester, MN, Mayo Clinic, 2 general internal medicine practices	100, Age 59 ± 16, 58% female	CBC (3 items)	91	2 (2.2)	2 (2.2)	
			Chemistry (12 items)	89	2 (2.2)	2 (2.2)	
			Lipids (3 items)	65	8 (12.3)	7 (9.3)	

Author	Setting	N	Test	No.	Diagnostic yield, n (%)	Therapeutic yield, n (%)	Comments
			Thyroid (either sTSH or T4) (5 items)	70	2 (2.8)	1 (1.5)	
			UA (5 items)	87	1 (1.1)	1 (1.1)	
			CBC (4 items)	325	5 (1.2)	3 (0.6)	
Boland et al., 1996	Rochester, MN, Mayo Clinic, four general internal medicine practices	531, Age 63 ± 14, 57% female	Chemistry panel (11 items)	289	12 (4.2)	8 (2.8)	50% of the yield due to glucose
			CBC (3 items)	266	49 (18.4)	44 (16.5)	
			Thyroid (either sTSH or T4) (3 items)	273	3 (1.1)	2 (0.7)	
			UA (5 items)	357	4 (1.1)	3 (0.8)	

*Yield of composite panel, expressing the percentage of patients who had the panel ordered for case-finding and had one or more new diagnoses (diagnostic yield) or one or more new diagnoses associated with change in management (therapeutic yield).

**ALT, alanine aminotransferase; UA, urinalysis; CBC, complete blood count.

light of differences in perceived value by patient and physicians, and differences in costs and reimbursable charges. In a larger prospective study conducted in four general internal medicine clinics, 531 patients had routine laboratory tests ordered for case-finding. The mean age of patients in this study was over 60 years. The overall diagnostic yield was 4.8% and the therapeutic yield was 4.0%. The therapeutic yield was 16.5% for the lipid panel, 2.8% for the chemistry panel, 0.9% for the complete blood count, 0.8% for urinalysis, and 0.7% for thyroid hormone test. Approximately half the therapeutic yield of the chemistry panel was due to the glucose. The therapeutic yield was not associated with age or gender, but was twice as high in new patients as in established patients (Boland et al., 1996). The Mayo Clinic patients were older than the patients studied in Basel, Switzerland, and would be expected to have a higher prevalence of disease, and the laboratory tests would be expected to have higher diagnostic and therapeutic yield. The studies from Switzerland and the United States are consistent in suggesting that, with the exception of the lipid panel, and possibly the serum glucose, laboratory tests for case-finding in ambulatory adults have a low (<1%) diagnostic and therapeutic yield.

The concept of the "annual physical examination" has evolved into the concept of the periodic health examination. There was little if any evidence of effectiveness of the annual physical examination in improving health outcomes (Charap, 1981). Largely based on the pioneering work of the Canadian Task Force on the Periodic Health Examination (CTPHE, 1976) and the U.S. Preventive Services Task Force (USPSTF, 1996), there is much better scientific basis for making decisions about laboratory testing for case-finding in the ambulatory setting. These interdisciplinary panels of experts have developed criteria for evaluating the evidence of the effectiveness of preventive services, including laboratory tests for case-finding (Table 5). The task force members and staff reviewed medical literature and made

Table 5   U.S. Preventive Services Task Force Rating System of Quality of Scientific Evidence

Level	Quality of Scientific Evidence
I	Evidence obtained from at least one properly designed randomized controlled trial.
II-1	Evidence obtained from well-designed controlled trials without randomization.
II-2	Evidence obtained from well-designed cohort or case-control analytic studies, preferably from more than one center or research group.
II-3	Evidence obtained from multiple time series with or without the intervention, or dramatic results in uncontrolled experiments (such as the results of the introduction of penicillin treatment in the 1940s).
III	Opinions of respected authorities, based on clinical experience, descriptive studies, or reports of expert committees

recommendations for preventive services for population-based demographic characteristics of populations at risk, the prevalence of disease, and evidence for the effectiveness of preventive services. Table 6 summarizes the recommendations of the U.S. Preventive Services Task Force for conditions for which laboratory tests are recommended for case-finding or screening.

ISSUES IN LABORATORY TESTS FOR CASE-FINDING

Need for Evidence for Effectiveness

There is extensive literature documenting inappropriate test ordering by physicians and methods to change physician test-ordering behavior (Solomon et al., 1998; Axt-Adam et al., 1993) A recent systematic overview of studies of laboratory use found that many studies that identify inappropriate laboratory use based on implicit or explicit criteria do not themselves meet methodologic standards suggested for audits of therapeutic maneuvers (van Walraven and Naylor, 1998; van Walraven et al., 1998). This may explain part of the wide variation in estimates of inappropriate laboratory test use.

Methodologic standards have been proposed for assessing the quality of diagnostic test evaluation (Mulrow et al., 1989). A recent review of methodologic standards in diagnostic test research was subtitled "Getting better but still not good." The study concluded that most diagnostic tests are still inadequately appraised. It suggested that predissemination evaluation of diagnostic tests could eliminate useless lab tests before they receive widespread application (Reid et al.,1995). The commonly available laboratory tests such as the complete blood count, chemistry profile, lipid panel, thyroid hormone tests, and urinalysis already have widespread application for the indication of case-finding. Ordering a test for case-finding is within the physicians' and other health providers' discretion. In the absence of evidence, there is a need for more attention to effectiveness before expanding the indications for a laboratory test from diagnosis and monitoring to the indication of case-finding in the ambulatory setting.

Problems in the Testing Cycle

A second issue relates to quality of care and laboratory tests. The Clinical Laboratory Improvement Amendments of 1988 (CLIA '88) focused attention on the laboratory's role in the quality of laboratory testing. As a result, there has been a substantial improvement in laboratory test performance. Recent studies suggest that now the majority of problems in the testing cycle occur in the preanalytic and postanalytic phases of testing. A study of laboratory testing in the primary-care setting was conducted in 49 practices in the Ambulatory Sentinel Practice Network (ASPN) and identified an occurrence rate of 1.1 problems per 1000 patient visits. Only 13% of problems, however, were attributed to the laboratory. Problems in test ordering and specimen handling were most common (56%); problems in the postanalytic

Table 6   U.S. Preventive Services Task Force Recommendations for Laboratory Tests for Case-Finding

Population group	Condition	Laboratory test	Recommendation
Birth to 10 years	Sickle-cell anemia	Hemoglobinopathy screen	At birth
	Phenylketonuria	Phenylalanine level	At birth
	Congenital hypothyroidism	T$_4$ and/or TSH	At birth
Ages 11–24 years	Cervical cancer	Papanicolaou (Pap) test	Female if sexually active at present
	Chlamydia	Chlamydia screen	Female >20 yr if sexually active
	Rubella	Rubella serology or vaccination history	Female >12 yr
Ages 25–64	Hypercholesterolemia	Total blood cholesterol	Men age 35–64, Women age 45–64
	Cervical cancer	Papanicolaou (Pap) test	Female annually
	Colorectal cancer	Fecal occult blood test	Annually
	Rubella	Rubella serology or vaccination history	Women of childbearing age
Age 65 and older	Colorectal cancer	Fecal occult blood test	Annually
	Cervical cancer	Papanicolaou (Pap) test	Female sexually active and have cervix
Pregnant women	Iron deficiency and other nutritional anemia	Hemoglobin/hematocrit	
	Hepatitis B	Hepatitis B surface antigen (HbsAg)	
	Syphilis	RPR/VDRL	
	Chlamydia	Chlamydia screen	<25 yr
	Rubella	Rubella serology or vaccination history	
	Newborn hemolysis	D (Rh) typing, antibody screen	
	Sickle-cell disease	Hemoglobinopathy screen	
	HIV	HIV screening	
	Urinary tract infection	Urine culture	12–16 wk
	Neural-tube defects	Serum α-fetoprotein	

phase were the next most frequent and occurred in 28% (Nutting et al., 1996). A second study of attending physicians and residents in medicine and internal medicine at a large urban teaching hospital and 21 affiliated suburban primary-care practices identified problems in ensuring that the results of tests ordered were received, problems in the notification of patients of the test results, and problems in the documentation of patient notification in medical records (Boohaker et al., 1996) It is reasonable to infer that these problems in the use of laboratory tests in general also occur when laboratory tests are used for case-finding in the ambulatory setting. Further studies of the quality of laboratory testing are needed with an emphasis on test ordering, result reporting, and patient notification documentation.

Genetic Testing

A third area is the impending development of a large number of new, expensive genetic tests that will emerge from the human genome project. Many of the currently available laboratory tests can detect phenotypic expression of genetic diseases. Genes have been identified for hemochromatosis, cystic fibrosis, muscular dystrophy, and other conditions and have been identified for a number of cancers including familial breast cancer and colorectal cancer. Our current practices for the diagnostic evaluation of suspected cases and testing family members are still being developed. The availability of new genetic tests will certainly accelerate more rapidly than our ability to evaluate the effectiveness of these tests in the ambulatory setting. Some of these tests will be used to confirm a diagnosis; many genetic tests, however, will be used for case-finding to detect disease in asymptomatic patients or predict future susceptibility to disease. Genetic tests will pose challenges to clinicians and laboratorians, based on concerns about ethical, legal, and social issues, as well as challenges in evaluating the effectiveness of these tests when used for case-finding.

Several aspects of genetic testing raise new issues that are different from the issues in the use of most of the commonly ordered tests currently used for case-finding in the ambulatory setting. One important aspect of genetic testing is that the tests are not always the criterion standard for establishing a diagnosis. Genetic testing can confirm the presence of mutations associated with disease. For some conditions the test is sufficient to confirm a diagnosis. For patients who are asymptomatic, the test provides a prediction of future occurrence of disease. Genetic tests for mutations associated with familial cancer, however, still have uncertainty in the prediction of risk over time for future cancer for patients with specific genetic mutations, as well as uncertainty in prediction of risk for patients without current detectable genetic mutation. There are no independent reference standards to validate genetic tests for future familial cancer, other than the future development of cancer. A second aspect of genetic testing that differs from most other routine tests is that the information from the test may affect the health care of relatives. A third aspect is that the information may affect decisions about reproduction. Current options for children and adults who are known to have positive genetic tests are highly variable, from no specific change in health care to intensive surveillance, pharmacotherapy, or surgery. A fourth aspect of genetic tests relates to ethical, legal, and social issues. Patients may encounter discrimination in insurance and employment, stigmatization, and experience psychological distress. A fifth aspect is that gene frequency differs by race and ethnicity, and there are racial and ethnic variations in access to health care and outcomes of health care. A sixth aspect is that most providers, laboratorians, and health-care workers have limited training in genetics, and there is an inadequate number of persons with training to provide genetic counseling. Clinicians and laboratorians and others interested in laboratory tests for case-finding will need to be aware of these issues as genetic tests become increasingly available.

SUMMARY

Laboratory tests are commonly used for case-finding in the ambulatory setting, despite evidence against their effectiveness in reducing death or disability and substantial evidence confirming the low diagnostic and therapeutic yield of these tests. Recent studies have shown that many routine preoperative tests are not effective in reducing postoperative complications, and guidelines for preoperative laboratory testing can reduce utilization and save resources. Similar studies have not been reported for routine laboratory testing in the ambulatory setting. It is quite likely that the growth in managed care will reduce utilization of low-yield tests that are not known to be effective. Although there are few quality-of-care problems in the testing cycle in the analytic phase of the testing cycle, there are quality problems in the preanalytic and the postanalytic phases of testing. Further efforts to improve quality of test ordering, result notification, and documentation of test result notification are needed. In the next few years there will be an explosion of genetic tests and increased focus on genetic tests for the case-finding in the ambulatory setting. Laboratorians and clinicians should be prepared to address these issues and should lead efforts to evaluate the effectiveness of laboratory tests and new genetic tests for case-finding and screening.

REFERENCES

Axt-Adam P, van der Wouden JC, van der Does E. Influencing behavior of physicians ordering laboratory tests: A literature study. *Med. Care* 1993;31:784–794.
Boland BJ, Wollan PC, Silverstein MD. Review of systems, physical examination, and routine tests for case–finding in ambulatory patients. *Am. J. Med. Sci.* 1995;309: 194–200.

Boland BJ, Wollan PC, Silverstein MD. Yield of laboratory tests for case-finding in the ambulatory general medical examination. *Am. J. Med.* 1996;101:142–152.

Boohaker EA, Ward RE, Uman JE, McCarthy BD. Patient notification and follow-up of abnormal test results. A physician survey. *Arch. Intern. Med.* 1996;156: 327–331.

Canadian Task Force on the Periodic Health Examination. The periodic health examination. *Can. Med. Asssoc. J.* 1979;1193–1254.

Charap MH. The periodic health examination: Genesis of a myth. *Ann. Intern. Med.* 1981;95:733–735.

Eisenburg JM, Myers LP, Pauly MV. How will changes in physician payment by Medicare influence laboratory testing? *JAMA* 1987;258:803–808.

Friedman GD, Collen MF, Fireman BH. Multiphasic Health Checkup Evaluation: A 16-year follow-up. *J. Chron. Dis.* 1986;39:453–463.

Kaplan EB, Sheiner LB, Boeckmann AJ, Roizen MF, Beal SL, Cohen SN, et al. The usefulness of preoperative laboratory screening. *JAMA* 1985;253:3576–3581.

Mulrow CD, Linn WD, Gaul MK, Pugh JA. Assessing quality of a diagnostic test evaluation. *J. Gen. Intern. Med.* 1989;4:288–295.

Nardella A, Pechet L, Snyder LM. Continuous improvement, quality control, and cost containment in clinical laboratory testing. Effects of establishing and implementing guidelines for preoperative tests. *Arch. Pathol. Lab. Med.* 1995;119: 518–522.

Narr BJ, Hansen TR, Warner MA. Preoperative laboratory screening in healthy Mayo patients: Cost-effective elimination of tests and unchanged outcomes. *Mayo Clin. Proc.* 1991;66:155–159.

Narr BJ, Warner ME, Schroeder DR, Warner MA. Outcomes of patients with no laboratory assessment before anesthesia and a surgical procedure. *Mayo Clin. Proc.* 1997;72:505–509.

Nutting PA, Main DS, Fischer PM, Stull TM, Pontious M, Seifert MJ, et al. Toward optimal laboratory use. Problems in laboratory testing in primary care. *JAMA* 1996;275:635–639.

Olsen DM, Kane RL, Proctor PH. A controlled trial of multiphasic screening. *N. Engl. J. Med.* 1976;294:925–930.

Ransohoff DF, Feinstein AR. Problems of spectrum and bias in evaluating the efficacy of diagnostic tests. *N. Engl. J. Med.* 1978;299:926–930.

Reid MC, Lachs MS, Feinstein AR. Use of methodological standards in diagnostic test research. Getting better but still not good. *JAMA* 1995;274:645–651.

Relman AS. Assessment and accountability: The third revolution in medical care [editorial]. *N. Eng. J. Med.* 1988;319:1220–1222.

Ruttimann S, Clemencon D. Usefulness of routine urine analysis in medical outpatients. *J. Med. Screening* 1994;1:84–87.

Ruttimann S, Clemencon D, Dubach UC. Usefulness of complete blood counts as a case-finding tool in medical outpatients. *Ann. Intern. Med.* 1992;116:44–50.

Ruttimann S, Dreifuss M, Clemencon D, di Gallo A, Dubach UC. Multiple biochemical blood testing as a case-finding tool in ambulatory medical patients [see comments]. *Am. J. Med.* 1993;94:141–148.

Silverstein MD. Decision making in clinical preventive medicine. *Primary Care Clin. Office Pract.* 1989;16:9–30.

Silverstein MD, Boland BJ. Conceptual framework for evaluating laboratory tests: Case-finding in ambulatory patients. *Clin. Chem.* 1994;40:1621–1627.

Solomon DH, Hashimoto H, Daltroy L, Liang MH. Techniques to improve physicians' use of diagnostic tests: A new conceptual framework. *JAMA* 1998;280: 2020–2027.

Turnbull JM, Buck C. The value of preoperative screening investigations in otherwise healthy individuals. *Arch. Intern. Med.* 1987;147:1101–1105.

U.S. Preventive Services Task Force. *Guide to Preventive Services*, second edition. Williams & Wilkins, Baltimore, 1996.

van Walraven C, Goel V, Chan B. Effect of population-based interventions on laboratory utilization: A time-series analysis. *JAMA* 1998;280:2028–2033.

van Walraven C, Naylor CD. Do we know what inappropriate laboratory utilization is? A systematic review of laboratory clinical audits. *JAMA* 1998;280:550–558.

Wilson JMG, Jungner G. *Principles and Practice of Screening for Disease*. World Health Organization, Geneva, 1968.

Chapter 10

Monitoring Patient Outcomes After Clinical Laboratory Testing

S. T. Mennemeyer, J. W. Winkelman, and C. I. Kiefe

This chapter describes a method of statistical investigation that we call *downstream event monitoring* (DEM), which looks at the population of patients who are tested by one or more clinical laboratories to discover adverse outcomes that may indicate a systematic problem. The problem may be specific to the laboratory, or it may be associated with equipment, reagents, testing practices, or patient characteristics. The approach attempts to use patient outcomes to monitor the accuracy of routine patient testing.

The accuracy of clinical laboratory testing has traditionally been monitored by the laboratory itself and by public regulators. A laboratory monitors itself with quality control sampling and techniques such as Shewhart chart graphing of test values (Shewhart, 1931). Regulators inspect a laboratory's equipment, operating procedures, and credentials of staff. In the United States, the Clinical Laboratory Improvement Act Amendments of 1988 (CLIA '88) required laboratories to be licensed and to participate in a program of proficiency testing if they perform tests of "moderate" or "high" complexity. The proficiency testing program challenges the laboratory to demonstrate its ability to correctly analyze a specially prepared sample that is sent to it without blinding. The current system does not monitor the accuracy of routine testing and processing of patient specimens (Shahangian, 1998).

Medicine today is being challenged to show how its practices are related to scientific evidence and to outcomes that are satisfactory to patients. Randomized controlled trials are now widely used to determine how well drugs, surgical procedures, and practice protocols work on specially selected samples of volunteers. Outcomes research, going a step further, examines what happens to the general population of patients when they are treated in different ways and whether what happens conforms to the patient's own wishes regarding survival and quality of life (USDHHS, 1991).

Clinical laboratories have not been leaders in the movement to study patient outcomes. One reason for this is the very practical problem of relating a laboratory test to an outcome when the test may be one of many things that are done to a patient during the process of diagnosis or treatment.

Nonetheless, a badly performed test may leave evidence. A false positive may produce a series of unnecessary follow up tests or treatments until the false result is detected. A false negative may leave a serious condition untreated until symptoms cannot be ignored or the patient dies. Tests that report the wrong value of some continuous measure may be followed by an event attributable to under or over dosage of an otherwise appropriate medication.

Alert clinicians do sometimes suspect that a laboratory test is wrong. They may order a retest. Comparison and investigation may reveal the original error. Retest orders are episodic responses to strong clinical suspicions. They may not alert a laboratory to a problem that affects their population of patients because individual clinicians who see a bad outcome for a single patient may dismiss it as an isolated occurrence not necessarily related to the laboratory's work. If the laboratory were aware of all of the adverse events seen by all of its clinicians, it might discover a problem that individual clinicians do not see.

HOW DOWNSTREAM EVENT MONITORING WORKS

Downstream event monitoring begins with a medical logic. It identifies a patient outcome that may be reasonably related to a prior laboratory test. For example, an outpatient prothrombin time (PT) test is often used by a physician to monitor the clotting speed of blood for a patient who is on anticoagulation therapy following either a stroke or a myocardial infarction. If the test reports an incorrect value, the physician may prescribe an inappropriate dosage of sodium warfarin (e.g., Coumadin). Too high a dose may promote bleeding either in the gastrointestinal tract or as a hemorrhagic stroke. Too low a dose may cause clotting that would produce either a thrombolytic stroke or a myocardial infarction. Thus a death or a hospitalization for a coagulation-related disorder is an adverse event that might be examined in relation to the PT test. Similarly, the serum digoxin test is used to measure the level of digoxin in the blood. Digoxin is a drug that affects the strength of the heart's pumping action. An inaccurate test result may encourage an inappropriate digoxin dosage adjustment. This implies that hospitalizations for various heartbeat irregularities might be examined for their relationship to prior laboratory testing. Similar logic would apply to almost any laboratory test that helps to regulate a medication dosage.

Another example would include the monitoring of glucose, triglycerides, and A1C for diabetics, where a hospitalization for diabetes-related disorders might result from problems with test accuracy. Similar logics have been developed for tests relating to cancer detection and urinary-tract infection (Mennemeyer and Winkelman, 1991).

Another key requirement for downstream monitoring is specification of a time period that elapses between when a test is performed and when the adverse event occurs. For the outpatient PT and serum digoxin tests, it may take a few days for a clinician to get back the test result, direct the patient to change the dosage, and achieve the desired level of medication in the blood. Adverse events within a few days of testing might thus be reasonably investigated for their relationship to the accuracy of a recent test. In contrast, inaccurate cholesterol testing may promote inadequate or overly aggressive efforts to lower cholesterol. It is unlikely, however, that a heart attack could reasonably be attributed to a recent cholesterol test except in cases where a medication reaction occurs.

DATA SOURCES

There are several data sources that might be used for downstream monitoring. Health insurance claims data in a fee-for-service setting have the advantage of being able to track patients from one provider to another according to dates of service. Thus, a hospital admission on Thursday can be related to a laboratory test on the previous Monday. Claims can also determine if the patient switched from using one lab to another or if other physicians became involved in the patient's care. Any switching of providers introduces opportunities for confusion and for changes in treatment that need to be considered in a statistical analysis. Claims can also track how frequently the patient had received a particular lab test prior to the index test. This allows one to control for the continuity of monitoring. The major disadvantage of claims data is that they contain limited clinical information. Diagnoses and procedures are coded, but the diligence and accuracy of this coding are driven by the documentation that an insurer requires for reimbursement purposes. The clinical findings of laboratory tests are, of course, not available in claims.

Studies of the accuracy of claims data have found them to be less detailed and reliable than medical records but nevertheless valuable for tracking utilization of services (Iezzoni et al., 1997). In some instances, claims data may prove more helpful than clinical records. For example, mammography and flu shots may be obtained by patients without any notation to this effect appearing in the medical record of the patient's regular physician (Melnikow and Kiefe, 1994).

Health maintenance organizations (HMOs), preferred provider organizations (PPOs), and other forms of managed care have become very interested in tracking the utilization of their members and maintaining sophisticated databases of patient encounters. This opens the possibility that outpatient laboratory tests can be related to subsequent adverse events.

Patient records offer the greatest detail about what tests were ordered, why they were ordered, and what they found. The main problem with them is that the patient record of one physician or one hospital generally does not contain information about the patient's use of another provider. The development of an electronic patient record that accumulates information about all providers would assist downstream event monitoring.

METHODS OF ANALYSIS

Analysis of downstream events needs to take account of the many variables that might influence a patient outcome. These variables include characteristics of the patient (e.g., demographics and comorbidities), the laboratory (e.g., size, ownership and staffing), and the physician (e.g., speciality). Logit analysis offers a convenient approach for exploring how these various independent variables affect the dependent variable, which is the probability that an adverse event occurs. In the logit model, the dependent variable may be simply a binary variable that equals 1 if the adverse event occurs and zero if it does not. Alternatively, the dependent variable could have multiple ("polytomous") categories such as heart attack, stroke, gastric bleeding, and no adverse event, as long as the categories can be defined to be mutually exclusive and exhaustive. When the binary dependent variable is used, the logit model is defined in terms of the logarithm of the odds that the adverse event occurs. Formally, this is:

$$\log[p/(1 - p)] = \exp(a + BX + CZ + DW)$$

where X, W, and Z are respectively vectors of variables for the characteristics of the patient, laboratory and physician; a, B, C, and D are vectors of coefficients; p is the probability that the adverse event occurs; and exp indicates the natural number e raised to the power in the parenthetic expression. The expression is generalized further when the dependent variable is polytomous. Maximum likelihood methods are used to fit the data to the logit expression (Hosmer & Lemeshow, 1989).

The coefficients of the logit model are used to produce conditional odds ratios that indicate how much the risk of an outcome is either increased or decreased relative to a baseline risk of 1.0 after taking account of the influence of the other variables in the model. A confidence region around the estimate is usually reported at the 95% level. For example, in one study we found that when a patient switched laboratories from one test to the next, the probability that a stroke would occur following the PT test was 1.57 times higher than if the patient had not switched laboratories. The 95% confidence region around this estimate was 1.31 to 1.89, indicating that it was quite likely that the estimated probability was above the baseline value of 1.0 (Mennemeyer and Winkelman, 1993).

The use of a logit model has both strengths and weaknesses for examining patient outcomes. A logit model estimates the probability that a particular test would have an adverse outcome given the characteristics of the patient on whom the test is performed, the lab doing that test, and the physician ordering the test. The logit model is thus an excellent tool for identifying individual "risk factors" in a sea of different variables. The simplicity of the logit model does, however, present some difficulties. It is generally cumbersome in logit analysis to control for fixed effects—such as the identity of each lab and each physician B that might exercise a common effect on a group of tests. This happens because there are usually many labs and many physicians in a database derived from claims data, and it is beyond the processing capabilities of computer programs to deal with the many dummy variables required to account for each one of these entities. One consequence of this complexity is that logit models often explain relatively little of the variance in patient outcomes, although they may identify some individual variables that are highly significant at influencing these outcomes. We discuss later some other data-mining techniques that may be helpful in addressing this problem.

APPLICATIONS

There have been two rounds of studies that examined the relation of adverse events to characteristics of laboratories and patients. The first round of studies examined Medicare Part A (i.e., hospital) and Part B (i.e., physician) claims for the period 1985–1987 for beneficiaries served by the Part B claim processing carriers for Delaware, Indiana, Pennsylvania, South Dakota, Washington, and the downstate portion of New York including New York City. (Mennemeyer & Winkelman, 1993; Winkelman and Mennemeyer, 1996a, 1996b) The second round also used Medicare claims for 1991 to 1993 for beneficiaries living in Alabama, Connecticut, Colorado, Iowa, Utah, and Wisconsin. In both rounds, the states were selected because they offered broad geographic diversity and because their data were to be linked to other economic or clinical studies (Pauly et al., 1991; Marciniak et al., 1998).

Both rounds have examined adverse events related to two separate tests: prothrombin time (PT) and serum digoxin. For either test, an adverse event is defined as a death or any hospitalization related to a specific list of conditions as defined by the International Classification of Diseases, Ninth Revision (ICD-9), or diagnosis-related group (DRG) codes found on Medicare Part A bills. For PT, the first round used conditions related to stroke (both thrombolytic and hemorrhagic), myocardial infarction, and sodium warfarin adverse drug reactions; the second round also included gastrointestinal bleeding. For digoxin, both rounds have used conditions related to hypertensive heart disease, congestive heart failure, and digoxin poisoning. For PT, the critical period of time following testing has been defined as 6 days with a 15-day period used to test the sensitivity of the results. For digoxin, the critical period has been defined as 15 days with sensitivity analysis at 30 days.

In both rounds, Part B claims were used to find all individuals who had received the outpatient test of interest and Part A claims were used to find all hospitalizations for the listed conditions. The A and B claims sets were then merged to link outpatient tests with subsequent hospitalizations. Medicare death records were used to find deaths in the relevant time periods. The claims were also used to measure several characteristics of beneficiaries and laboratories in reference to the date of any index test. These included the number of tests received by the beneficiary up to 6 months prior to the index test; the number of tests performed by the laboratory on the index date and up to 6 months before the date; whether a different laboratory had performed an immediately prior test; and the amount paid by Medicare on behalf of the beneficiary for outpatient and inpatient care for up to 6 months before the index date.

The first round of studies found the following.

1. Physician office laboratories (POLs) that perform less than 40 PT tests per month have probabilities of adverse events that are about 2 to 3 times higher than commercial laboratories. No small lab effect was found for digoxin. The more automated equipment used at that time for digoxin testing may explain this finding.

2. The probability of an adverse event is reduced for PT tests when beneficiaries have a history of prior testing; prior testing did not matter for digoxin testing. The more complex and less standardized reporting format for PT results used at that time may explain this result.

3. Switching from one laboratory to another increases the probability of an adverse event by about 14% (for digoxin) up to 57% (for PT). Discontinuity in care or confusion from differences in reporting formats among laboratories may explain this result.

4. Relative to New York, tests performed in other states had probabilities of adverse events that were up to twice as high; this result was more pronounced for PT than for digoxin. New York's strong inspection program may explain this finding.

5. Sicker patients, as indicated by their history of prior Medicare spending, had higher probabilities of adverse events.

Second-round studies are still in progress. One issue of continuing interest is the various ways of defining an adverse event and the relation of these events to the type of laboratory. Table 1 shows, for example, the frequency of adverse events following PT testing by type of laboratory for the six states in the round two study of PT. Here events within 6 days of testing were classified into four categories. "Undercoagulation" events are those where the diagnoses or procedure codes clearly suggest a problem of hemorrhaging that would be consistent with undercoagulation of the blood. Diagnosis codes such as intracerebral hemorrhage, subdural hemorrhage, gastric ulcer with hemorrhage, and gastrointestinal hemorrhage are examples. "Overcoagulation" events are those where a clotting problem is evident, such as cerebrovascular embolism and phlebitis. A third category consists of acute

Table 1   Frequency of Adverse Events Following PT Testing by Type of Laboratory, 1991–1993, Six States

Laboratory type	AMI & other[a]	Undercoagulation[b]	Overcoagulation[c]	No adverse event	Total
Commercial	3,652	1,579	3,609	1,192,575	1,201,415
	(0.30%)	(0.13%)	(0.30%)	(99.26%)	(100%)
POL	2,090	1,504	3,928	1,053,104	1,060,626
	(0.20%)	(0.14%)	(0.37%)	(99.29%)	(100%)
Hospital OPD	9,339	2,220	5,546	1,401,578	1,418,683
	(0.66%)	(0.16%)	(0.39%)	(98.79%)	(100%)
Total	15,081	5,303	13,083	3,647,257	3,680,724
	(0.41%)	(0.14%)	(0.36%)	(99.09%)	(100%)

Note. Reject null hypothesis that outcomes are the same by type of laboratory, chi-square = 3847, df = 6, p = .001. Source: Author's computations, see text.

[a]ICD-9-C codes 410.0 through 410.9 "acute myocardial infarction," 411.81 "coronary occlusion without MI," 286 through 286.99 with E858.2 "Coagulation Defects."

[b]ICD-9-CM codes 431 intracerebral hemorrhage, 432.0 nontraumatic extradural hemorrhage, 432.1 subdural hemorrhage, 432.9 unspecified intracranial hemorrhage, 459 hemorrhage unspecified, 531.0/2/4/6 gastric ulcer (with various hemorrhage &/or perforation), 532.0/2/4/6 duodenal ulcer (with various hemorrhage &/or perforation), 562.02/03 diverticulosis of small intestine with hemorrhage, 562.12/13 diverticulosis of colon with hemorrhage, 578 (all subcategories) gastrointestinal hemorrhage, 786.3 hemoptysis (cough with hemorrhage, pulmonary hemorrhage not elsewhere classified), 965.2 poisoning by agents...anticoagulants.

[c]433 to 436.99 occulsions & stenosis of precerebral arteries, 434.1 cerebrovascular embolism, 444 (all subcategories) arterial embolism and thrombosis, 451.1 phlebitis and thrombophlebitis...lower extremities, 451.83 phlebitis and thrombophlebitis...upper extremities, other 451s phlebitis and thrombophlebitis, 452 (all subcategories) portal vein thrombosis, 453.3/8/9 other venulous embolism and thrombosis (various sites).

myocardial infarction and various other coagulation defects that do not clearly belong in the previous overcoagulation and undercoagulation categories. The fourth category is "No Adverse Event,"—that is, the beneficiary did not experience a death or a hospitalization related to a coagulation problem.

The table shows that adverse events following PT testing are fairly rare. All three categories of adverse events total to 33,467, which is slightly less than 1% of the total 3.6 million PT tests. Nonetheless, there is enough variation among adverse event categories and types of laboratories to reject the null hypothesis that the frequency of events is independent of laboratory type. In particular, hospital outpatient departments seem to have more tests followed by adverse events, especially AMI and other coagulation defects. This may reflect characteristics of either the patients themselves or the laboratories (Mennemeyer et al., 1999).

We estimated a logit model, similar to the model that was estimated in the first round of studies. The model controlled for beneficiary demographics (age, race, sex), previous Medicare spending for outpatient and inpatient services, the number of tests, if any, received by the beneficiary in the prior

6 months, state of residence, and membership in an HMO. Laboratory characteristics included in the model were the daily and monthly volume of Medicare tests for PT. These variables controlled for any effect of volume on proficiency. The model also controlled for whether or not the test was performed on a weekend because this might affect the seriousness of the patient's condition as well as whether or not the laboratory was open for business. Table 2 shows the resulting conditional odds ratios. Relative to tests performed in a commercial laboratory, tests performed in POLs have a lower probability of being followed by an adverse event. For myocardial infarctions and other coagulation defects, the probability is only 0.28, compared to 1.0 for the commercial laboratory—that is, slightly more than 70% lower. The 95% confidence region around this estimate is .25 to .33. Because the confidence region remains below the reference value of 1.0 for commercial laboratories, it would be judged statistically significant. Similar remarks apply to Undercoagulation and Overcoagulation categories, where the odds ratios for POLs are respectively .71 (95% CI .59 to .85) and .61 (95% CI .54 to .70). For hospital outpatient department laboratories (OPDs) the story is a bit more complicated. Test performed in OPDs have a higher probability of being followed by MIs and coagulation defects and a slightly lower probability of being followed by undercoagulation and overcoagulation events.

Table 2 also shows, in brackets, the simple odds ratios that could be computed directly from Table 1. For example, the simple odds ratio for an adverse event due to overcoagulation for a POL relative to a commercial laboratory is 1.23 [i.e., (3928/1,060,626)/(3609/1,201,415)]. The simple ratio suggests that patients tested in POLs have a 23% higher probability of experiencing an adverse event related to overcoagulation relative to a commercial laboratory. However, once the model adjusts for the other characteristics of the patient and laboratory, the odds ratio falls to .62, showing that physician ownership of the laboratory, by itself, is associated with a lower

Table 2 Conditional Odds Ratios (95% Confidence Intervals in Parentheses) for Adverse Events by Type of Laboratory [Simple Odds Ratio in Brackets]

Laboratory type	AMI & other[a]	Undercoagulation[b]	Overcoagulation[c]
Commercial	1.0	1.0	1.0
POL	.28	.71	.62
	(.25 to .33)	(.59 to .85)	(.54 to .70)
	[.65]	[1.08]	[1.23]
Hospital OPD	1.22	.78	.93
	(1.16 to 1.29)	(.71 to .85)	(.88 to .98)
	[2.17]	[1.20]	[1.31]

Source: Author's computations from Medicare Claims 1991–1993, see text.
[a,b,c]Defined in Table 1.

risk of an adverse event. This illustrates the importance of adjusting for as many relevant characteristics as possible, and it invites questions about how other characteristics of the laboratory such as its equipment and personnel might affect these outcomes.

Under CLIA '88 licensure procedures, commercial laboratories and physician office laboratories (POLs) were required to complete Health Care Financing Administration (HCFA) Form 109. The form requires the laboratory to identify the equipment and reagents used in performing specific tests. The form also asks about the educational and professional credentials of personnel who direct the laboratory and supervise or perform tests. For round two studies, a sample of laboratories was selected and their Form 109 information was retrieved. This allows analysis of the effects of equipment, reagents, and personnel on adverse events. This analysis is still in progress, but our preliminary analyses suggest that adverse events may be less frequent in POLs relative to commercial laboratories. This may be due to the decision of small POLs to stop performing the PT due to the tougher CLIA '88 licensure requirements.

OTHER APPROACHES

Other investigators have been developing different approaches to monitor the accuracy of routine laboratory testing. One proposed approach is to combine classification and regression tree analysis (CART) with a logit model (Steinberg and Cardell, 1999). CART is a data analysis technique that sorts data into nodes (e.g., all labs in Alabama owned by physicians; patients over age 85 who had no prior tests) that are highly associated with a particular outcome. Often these nodes have no obvious analytical meaning. The number of nodes discovered by CART is likely, however, to be much fewer than the number of potential fixed effects. Some of these nodes might be individual laboratories or individual physicians that have a high probability of generating adverse events. The proposed approach is to include the CART nodes as dummy variables in the logit model. This would help to discover the risk factors associated with the general characteristics of patients, laboratories, and physicians after controlling for risk-prone nodes.

Elsewhere in this volume, Moser and Brossette describe a rule-based data-mining approach that uses hospital inpatient clinical laboratory data to discover outbreaks of infection, drug resistance, and other adverse events. A rule-based system checks continuously for sequences and correlations that depart from the standard experience. For example, the system is supposed to discover a sudden rise in the frequency of an antibiotic resistance in the cardiac intensive care unit. The aim of the approach is to develop a method of data analysis that would allow an institution to find problems within a few days of an outbreak that might otherwise go undetected for weeks. At present a group of clinical experts in the institution has to examine the statistical output to decide what merits further investigation. As the system accumulates experience, it may be possible to fine-tune it to require less input from the clinical staff. In principle, the approach could be applied to multiple institutions using a pooled database. There is no philosophical difference between rule-based data mining and downstream event monitoring. The two approaches have simply focused on different data sets, institutional settings, and statistical techniques.

Split-sample testing is another approach for checking the accuracy of routine testing. Shahangian and colleagues report on two demonstrations where patient specimens were split and sent it to multiple laboratories. One demonstration involved testing for serum total cholesterol (n = 646) and potassium (n = 732) at 11 medical clinics evaluating 30 to 199 patients. Clinical personnel collected three tubes of blood from each patient (Shahangian et al., 1998a). One specimen was processed routinely, the second was sent to a reference laboratory, and a third "audit" specimen was sent to a storage facility. When results were sufficiently discrepant between the routine and reference laboratories, the audit sample was split into three parts; the first two were sent back to the original laboratories and the third went to a referee laboratory. A random selection of audit samples was also sent out in this manner. Using a three-criteria statistical method, the discrepancy rates were 2.8% to 8.7% for potassium and 1.5% to 4.6% for cholesterol. A second demonstration had a similar design to examine discrepancy in results for serum potassium, serum total cholesterol, and whole-blood hemoglobin on 177 patients in nine clinics (Shahangian et al., 1998b).

The split-sample approach has the merit of examining discrepancies in testing on routine patient specimens. Potentially, it offers a much clearer picture of a laboratory's testing performance compared to proficiency testing, which usually uses specially prepared specimens. Splitting samples poses practical difficulties of coordination plus higher expense simply from doing tests in parallel. Statistical methods for comparing results among laboratories also pose problems because of the physical restrictions on how much material can be obtained from one person that can be split among multiple laboratories. Despite these difficulties, however, the technique is very promising.

COST-EFFECTIVENESS

The potential cost-effectiveness of downstream event monitoring, data mining, and sample splitting have not yet been determined. Research has focused on whether any of these methods can find events that are sufficiently suspicious to warrant further investigation. Whether subsequent investigations would find real and correctable testing problems that would in turn reduce patient hospitalizations and death is unknown. The different techniques clearly differ in terms of their fixed and variable costs. Downstream event monitoring is largely a fixed-cost activity in the sense that most of its expense involves building a database, which can then be analyzed with little additional cost as the number of laboratories, tests, or beneficiaries increases in the database. Rule-based data mining involves the fixed costs of setting up a data system plus ongoing costs as experts continually update and evaluate its output. Both approaches are thus likely to have large economies of scale. Sample splitting involves some organizational set-up costs, but most of its expenses come from multiple testing of a given patient, and thus it would probably have fewer economies of scale.

A rough estimate of the cost savings that might be achieved from downstream event monitoring of prothrombin time testing is the following. Using Medicare claims in six states for 1991–1993, there were 33,467 adverse events subsequent to 3,680,724 tests. A conservative estimate of the cost saving from avoiding a bad event is the average cost of a hospitalization, which was $6,262 in 1995 (American Hospital Association, 1997). This is conservative because it ignores rehabilitation and nursing home costs following a stroke or myocardial infarction and it pretends that a death is "worth" only the cost of a hospitalization. A 10% reduction in the number of bad events would thus be worth roughly $20 million (i.e., $33,467 \times 0.10 \times 6262$). Database construction and analysis for downstream events in an academic research setting have been below $500,000 for a cost savings per research dollar ratio of about 42 to 1. Research costs are probably higher than would be the costs of retrieving and analyzing data on an ongoing basis. The figures here are obviously speculative, but the point is that data monitoring costs are fairly cheap compared to the expense of the events that might be prevented.

CONCLUSIONS

From several different perspectives, techniques are being developed to examine the accuracy of clinical laboratory testing by looking at the results of routine daily testing and what happens to patients after testing. In the not-too-distant future, clinical laboratories are likely to be linked together to share their data and possibly a sample of patient specimens. Statistical analysis may compare the results reported by different laboratories for a test done on the same day for the same patient. Patients may also be tracked statistically to see if they experience unusual frequencies of adverse events that might indicate a laboratory problem. This is a considerable advance beyond the customary approaches of inspection and proficiency testing.

The speed of development and adoption of new systems of laboratory test monitoring will depend upon their perceived benefit from saving lives, preventing hospitalizations, and, ultimately, reducing costs.

ACKNOWLEDGMENTS

Support for the author's research has been provided by the U.S. Department of Health and Human Services, Office of Health Policy, Assistant Secretary for Planning and Evaluation, under contract HHS-100-89-0017 to Abt Associates, Inc., Cambridge, MA, and by the U.S. Centers for Disease Control and Prevention under cooperative agreement S010-13/13, "Evaluation of Laboratory Performance and Practice Data to Guide Interventions to Improve Quality of Laboratory Practice," with the Association of Schools of Public Health and the School of Public Health, University of Alabama at Birmingham. The author thanks project officers Herb Hammond, George Greenburg, and Steven Steindel for their advice and encouragement. Views expressed are solely the author's.

REFERENCES

American Hospital Association. Hospital Statistics (annual) as reproduced in U.S. Department of Commerce, *Statistical Abstract of the United States*, Table 188, p. 129, 1997.

Hosmer DW Jr, Lemeshow S. *Applied Logistic Regression Analysis*. John Wiley and Sons, New York, 1989.

Iezzoni LI (ed.). *Risk Adjustment for Measuring Healthcare Outcomes*, second edition. Health Administration Press, Chicago, 1997.

Marciniak TA, Ellerbeck EF, Radford MJ, Kresowik TF, Gold JA, Krumholz HM, Kiefe CI, Allman RM, Vogel RA, Jencks SF. Improving the quality of care for Medicare patients with acute myocardial infarction: Results from the Cooperative Cardiovascular Project. *JAMA* 1998;279(17):13517.

Mennemeyer ST, Winkelman JW. Downstream outcomes: Using insurance claims data to screen for errors in clinical laboratory testing. *Qual. Rev. Bull.* 1991;17(6)194–199.

Mennemeyer ST, Winkelman JW. Searching for inaccuracy in clinical laboratory testing using Medicare data: Evidence for prothrombin time. *JAMA* 1993;269(8):1030–1033.

Mennemeyer ST, Winkelman JW, Kiefe CI. Effect of Laboratory Equipment and Personnel on Patient Outcomes Following Prothrombin Time Testing. Invited paper, Academy of Clinical Laboratory Physicians and Scientists, Salt Lake City, UT, June 1999.

Melnikow J, Kiefe C. Patient compliance and medical research: Issues in methodology. *J. Gen. Intern. Med.* 1994;9(2):96105.

Pauly MV, Mennemeyer ST, Eisenberg JM, Reardon LR. Assessment of the Effects of Reimbursement Policy on the Utilization of Clinical laboratory Testing and the Propensity of Physicians to Perform In-Office Testing. Abt Associates, Inc., Cambridge, MA, Contract HHS-100-89-0017, 1991.

Shahangian S. Proficiency testing in laboratory medicine: Uses and limitations. *Arch. Pathol. Lab. Med.* 1998;122(1):1530.

Shahangian S, Cohn RD, Gaunt EE, Krolak JM. System to monitor a portion of the total testing process in medical clinics and laboratories: Evaluation of a split-specimen design. *Clin. Chem.* 1998a;45(2):26980.

Shahangian S, Krolak JM, Gaunt EE, Cohn RD. A system to monitor a portion of the total testing process in medical clinics and laboratories: Feasibility of a splitspecimen design. *Arch. Pathol. Lab. Med.* 1998b;122(6):50311.

Shewhart WA. *Economic Control of Quality of Manufactured Product*. D. Van Nostrand, New York, 1931, republished in 1980 by the American Society for Quality Control, Milwaukee, WI.

Steinberg DN, Cardell NS. *The Hybrid CART-Logit Model in Classification and Data Mining*. Salford Systems, San Diego, CA, 1999.

U.S. Department of health and Human Services (USDHHS) Public Health Service, Agency for Health Care Policy and Research. *Research Activities*, No. 138, February 1991.

Winkelman JW, Mennemeyer ST. Screening for clinical laboratory errors with Medicare claims data: Results for digoxin. *Am. J. Med. Qual.* 1996a;11(1):25–32.

Winkelman JW, Mennemeyer S. Using patient outcomes to screen for clinical laboratory errors. *Clin. Lab. Manage. Rev.* 1996b;10(2):134–142.

Chapter 11

Outcomes Management in Anatomic Pathology

S. S. Raab

In anatomic pathology, outcomes analysis is not new, but has been very focused. For years, the anatomic pathology literature, scientific meetings, and discussion have been centered on patient outcomes as the ultimate goal or the endpoint of medical care. Anatomic pathologists may not view themselves as active participants in outcomes analysis, but much of what anatomic pathologists do is to produce data that are used to affect patient care. In anatomic pathology, data comes in the form of the "diagnosis," and anatomic pathology departments serve as the gatekeepers of valuable medical information (Raab et al., 1994a).

Perfecting pathologic diagnoses presumably improves patients' outcomes, such as survival and quality of life. This is well illustrated, for example, in the area of breast pathology. For the past several decades, the anatomic pathology literature has focused on classification of breast lesions, recognition of potential pitfalls in diagnosis, and the application of ancillary tools, such as immunohistochemistry, to aid in diagnostic decision making, There are different diagnostic "camps," which believe that their diagnostic schema are more predictive or more useful than other diagnostic schema (Page and Simpson, 1999; Page and Dupont, 1998; Page et al., 1998; Rosen, 1993; Rosen et al., 1995; Fisher, 1997; Fisher et al., 1998; Fechner, 1993; Schnitt, 1998). According to the data produced by some researchers, such as Page et al., women have a different risk to develop invasive breast cancer depending on the classification of their breast disease (Page et al., 1998; Page and Dupont, 1998; Page and Simpson, 1999). Breast fine needle aspiration (FNA) and core biopsy have blossomed because these techniques are believed to be extremely accurate in providing diagnostic information and less costly and invasive compared to other diagnostic tests such as open biopsy (Raab et al., 1994a; Page and Simpson, 1999; Page and Dupont, 1998; Page et al., 1998; Rosen, 1993; Rosen et al., 1995; Fisher, 1997; Fisher et al., 1998;

Fechner, 1993; Schnitt, 1998; Sanchez and Stahl, 1996; Boerner et al., 1999; Ellis and Pinder, 1998; Snead et al., 1997; Boerner and Sneige, 1998; Layfield et al., 1993). Immunohistochemical markers such as the estrogen and progesterone receptor proteins and the c-erbB-2 (HER-2/neu) protein are thought to be useful because they may predict the clinical response to specific therapeutic approaches (Makris et al., 1997; Ross and Fletcher, 1998; Yang et al., 1999). Thus, these immunostains may serve as prognostic indicators and be able to predict the survival of a patient population (Wick et al., in press). All of these studies and advancements in breast pathology are patient-outcome centered because they improve or refine diagnoses and treatment options, thus improving patient care.

The chapter focuses on some of the better-studied areas of patient outcomes management from the anatomic laboratory perspective.

MEASURES OF ANATOMIC PATHOLOGY TEST PERFORMANCE

Clinicians and pathologists often have contrasting views as to how anatomic pathology diagnoses should be used in patient care. Some clinicians argue for a Bayesian approach, in which the anatomic pathology diagnosis is interpreted probabilistically and used to calculate the posttest probability of disease from the pretest probability of disease (Schwartz et al., 1981; Sackett et al., 1991; Raab et al., 1995). For example, if a bronchoscopic biopsy of a peri-hilar lung mass is performed, the pathologic diagnosis could be interpreted as 95% probable non-small cell carcinoma and 5% probable granulomatous disease, rather than the traditional diagnoses of "non-small cell carcinoma" or "granuloma" (Schwartz et al., 1981). This probabilistic approach allows for clinicians to integrate their clinical impressions with the pathologic diagnosis in individual scenarios. Many pathologists argue against using this approach because they think that it is unnatural to report diagnoses in a probabilistic manner and that the majority of clinicians act, at best, only in a quasi-Bayesian fashion (Raab et al., 1995). In the more traditionalist nonprobabilistic approach, pathologists and clinicians often view diagnoses as right or wrong. This has led to the use of accuracy measures such as sensitivity, specificity, positive predictive value, and negative predictive value to describe test performance (Raab, 1994; Sackett et al., 1991). Most articles in the anatomic pathology literature have used these measures to investigate test accuracy (Raab et al., 1994a). Measuring accuracy is important from the patient outcomes perspective because it allows clinicians to know how and when to use certain diagnostic tests (Sackett et al., 1991).

The problem with using measures such as sensitivity and specificity is that these measures cannot be used in a given clinical scenario (e.g., even if the test sensitivity is 98%, one cannot know if any given test is a true or false positive) (Raab, 1994; Sackett et al., 1991). A second problem is that sensitivity and specificity are best suited for binary diagnoses (e.g., the diagnosis is either benign or malignant), and many anatomic pathology diagnoses are not binary (Raab, 1994; Sackett et al., 1991). This is most apparent in the field of cytology, where it is not infrequent to use the more qualitative diagnoses of atypical, suspicious, or probably malignant (Raab, 1994). The reporting of diagnoses qualitatively is, of course, one of the main reasons why clinicians argue for the probabilistic approach. There is validity in the question of how one treats a patient who has "probable" cancer (Schwartz et al., 1991; Raab et al., 1995). The answer is to use other measures of accuracy such as likelihood ratios (LRs) and receiver operating characteristic (ROC) curves, which are able to effectively deal with nonbinary diagnoses, thus still allowing pathologists to use qualitative diagnoses (Raab, 1994; Sackett et al., 1991; Radack et al., 1986; Giard and Hermans, 1990; Langley et al., 1985; Beck and Shultz, 1986; McNeil and Ranley, 1984).

During the past several decades, anatomic pathology articles have demonstrated the benefits of LRs from the patient perspective (Sackett et al., 1991, Radack et al., 1986; Giard and Hermans, 1990). LRs may be calculated for individual diagnostic categories (e.g., an LR for benign and an LR for probably cancer) and allow clinicians to operate in a Bayesian manner to calculate posttest probabilities from individual pathologic diagnoses (Raab, 1994; Sackett et al., 1991). In the pathology literature, LRs have been effectively calculated for bronchial brush and breast fine needle aspiration specimens (Raab et al., 1995; Radack et al., 1986; Giard and Hermans, 1990). LRs show the problem with thinking in black and white diagnostic terms and also that individual pathologists have different certainties when they use diagnoses such as suspicious (Raab, 1994).

ROC curves have been more extensively used in radiology and clinical pathology than in anatomic pathology (Ranley and McNeil, 1982; Metz, 1986). In anatomic pathology, ROC curves may be used to calculate diagnostic accuracy of qualitative diagnostic schema (Raab et al., 1995; Raab, 1994; Toogood, 1980; Radack et al., 1986; Giard and Hermans, 1990; Langley et al., 1985; Renshaw et al., 1997). For example, ROC curves could calculate the accuracy of bronchial brush specimens in diagnosing malignancy even if a cytology laboratory used diagnoses such as atypical or possible cancer (Raab et al., 1995). ROC curves have proven to be effective in outcomes management because they may be used to compare diagnostic accuracy in different clinical scenarios (Raab et al., 1995; Cohen et al., 1987; Liu et al., 1999; Oweity et al., 1998). For example, in the interpretation of breast FNAs, ROC curve analysis has shown that more experienced pathologists are more accurate than less experienced pathologists (Cohen et al., 1987). Using ROC curve analysis, Liu et al. (1999) and Oweity et al. (1998) showed that specimens with clinical history could be more accurately interpreted than specimens without clinical history. This indicates that there potentially may be more diagnostic "errors" if clinical history is not provided on specimen requisition forms.

These forms of statistical accuracy analysis have helped to elucidate the role of the pathologic diagnosis in overall patient care. The motivations of the clinical staff who obtain diagnostic tests and the actual impact and meaning of pathologic diagnoses are increasingly being studied. For example, many clinicians do not understand that the autopsy serves as an important quality assurance tool for all of medical practice (Veress and Alafuzoff, 1993, 1994; Szende et al., 1996; Stevanovic et al., 1986; Landefeld et al., 1988; Burton et al., 1998; dePangher et al.,1995; Sarode et al., 1993; Grundmann, 1994). It is estimated that there is a major discrepancy between the clinical premortem diagnosis and the postmortem diagnosis in greater than 30% of all cases in which an autopsy is performed (Sarode et al., 1993). This percentage has remained unchanged (Burton et al., 1998) despite advances in technology and diagnosis, and this has profound implications for medical care cost and quality. In a United Kingdom survey (Karunaratne and Benbow, 1997), 11.3% of clinicians thought that the autopsy consisted of "unacceptable mutilation." This emphasizes the concept that clinicians who order pathologic tests may not understand the biases, benefits, or limitations of these tests.

For example, in working up patients with radiographically detected lung masses, pulmonologists accurately estimate the diagnostic accuracy of bronchoscopy but underestimate the diagnostic accuracy of other tests, such as sputum cytology (Raab et al., 1999c). On the other hand, primary care physicians often choose sputum cytology and transthoracic FNA as the first tests to order in patients with potential lung tumors (Burton et al., 1998). In a university setting, Steffee et al. (1997) showed that the number of sputum cytology specimens markedly decreased in the past decade and that bronchoscopic (with transbronchial FNA) specimens increased (Steffee et al., 1997; Fraire et al., 1991). This may be due to the fact that if patients with lung lesions presented at this university, they were immediately referred to the pulmonology division and bronchoscopy was performed. Preferential test ordering has a marked impact on several aspects of patient care (Morretin, 1989; Cooncy, 1992; Berenson, 1986; Schroeder and Showstack, 1978; Epstein et al., 1984; Eisenburg et al., 1987), such as cost-effectiveness. The use of high-technology tests and preferential test ordering have been considered to be contributing causes for the rising costs of health care (Morretin, 1989; Cooncy, 1992; Berenson, 1986; Schroeder and Showstack, 1978).

INTEROBSERVER VARIABILITY

Because pathology diagnoses are subjective, there is an inherent interobserver diagnostic variability, meaning that even if pathologists examine the same microscopic fields, they may disagree about the diagnosis (Raab et al., 1994a). Studies measuring interobserver diagnostic variability have been performed in almost all areas of anatomic pathology (Raab et al., 1994a). In some instances, interobserver diagnostic variability is a reflection of pathologists using different diagnostic criteria; at other times it is a reflection of experience or skill (Raab et al., 1994a). The measure of interobserver diagnostic variability is clinically important if differences in diagnosis actually affect patient care. Any degree of interobserver diagnostic variability may create the perception that there is a lack of a true gold standard diagnosis (Schwartz et al., 1981), which serves as a basis for much of medical treatment. Interobserver diagnostic variability often is incorrectly interpreted by both pathologists and clinicians as diagnostic error (Foucar, 1997, 1998; Nakleh and Zarbo, 1998; Frable, 1997; Kreiger, 1997; Hocking et al., 1997; Safrin and Bark, 1993; Goldstein, in press), which is discussed later in this chapter. A portion of interobserver diagnostic variability is due to differences in opinion (Raab et al., 1994a).

One of the more well-quoted and important studies in interobserver diagnostic variability was performed by Rosai (1991), who presented preselected microscopic fields of breast lesions to expert breast pathologists. In some of the cases, the expert pathologists demonstrated a large degree of interobserver diagnostic variability, with some pathologists making benign diagnoses and other pathologists making malignant diagnoses. These differences in opinion not only would affect patient care in these individual circumstances, but also would affect the perceptions related to specific disease processes. For example, if a malignant diagnosis is "overused" in one institution (i.e., many truly benign lesions are diagnosed as malignant), the follow-up for patients with a malignant diagnosis at that institution would be skewed (e.g., patients with a malignant diagnosis would do better than patients at other institutions that did not overuse a malignant diagnosis) (Raab et al., 1997b).

In the area of cervical vaginal cytology, interobserver diagnostic variability studies have shown poor correlation among observers, particularly when they examine "atypical" smears (Hocking et al., 1997; Foucar, 1997; Safrin and Bark, 1993; Goldstein, in press; Rosai, 1991; Raab et al., 1997b; Confortini et al., 1993; Young et al., 1994; Yobs et al., 1987; Sherman et al., 1992, 1994; O'Sullivan, 1998). Raab et al. showed that four expert cytologists seldom agreed on which retrospectively reviewed Pap smears should be diagnosed as atypical glandular cells of undetermined significance (AGUS) (Raab et al., 1998a). The mean kappa statistic for pairwise cytopathologist comparison varied from 0.16 to 0.27, indicating poor agreement (Raab et al., 1998a). This interobserver diagnostic variability has clinical implications, because the American Society for Colposcopy and Cervical Cytology recommends that all women who have an AGUS diagnosis receive aggressive follow-up (e.g., colposcopy with biopsy and curettage) (Cox, 1997). Given the reportedly high number of women with AGUS who have clinically significant lesions on follow-up, this recommendation may be valid, but it is unlikely that all institutions use the AGUS diagnosis in the same way (Raab et al., 1998a). What some pathologists call AGUS, others call benign (and vice versa), indicating that cases that are called AGUS in some laboratories are potentially missed in other laboratories. This level of diagnostic disagreement has medical implications, because "expert" pathologists will testify that certain smears were "misdiagnosed," rather than arguing that differences in diagnosis were related to interobserver diagnostic variability. The fallacy is that, at least for AGUS diagnoses, expert pathologists do not agree anyway and the AGUS category is poorly understood. Performing interobserver diagnostic variability studies helps to identify the areas in pathology that lack well-defined diagnostic criteria, which may be targeted in future studies (Raab et al., 1994a).

Although interobserver diagnostic variability may never be completely eliminated, decreasing interobserver diagnostic variability is a goal of many pathologists. One method to decrease interobserver diagnostic variability has been to teach pathologists the diagnostic criteria of an expert or the consensus criteria derived from a group of experts (Schnitt et al., 1992; Scott et al., 1997; Dalton et al., 1994; Raab et al., 1996, 1997a). In a follow-up study of atypical breast lesions, Schnitt et al. (1992) showed that if pathologists were given a specific list of criteria, interobserver diagnostic variability decreased. Statistical analysis has been used to determine the optimal criteria for diagnosis and these criteria have been used to educate pathologists. This statistical method has been used most extensively in cytology. For example, Raab et al. (1994b) used logistic regression analysis to determine the most sensitive and specific criteria to separate low-grade transitional-cell carcinomas from reactive lesions in bladder wash specimens; after a teaching session, pathologists successfully used these criteria in a second study to classify unknown bladder wash specimens (Raab et al., 1996). The practice of sending difficult cases to expert pathologists is thought to decrease interobserver diagnostic variability and error (Abt et al., 1995; Silverberg, 1995). Some specialists advocate this approach despite the increase in medical care expenses. In a gynecologic pathology study, the detection of errors through expert review was thought to justify the extra cost (Santoso et al., 1998).

Increasing diagnostic standardization is a separate issue but related to interobserver diagnostic variability. One example of diagnostic standardization is the implementation of the Bethesda system diagnostic categories for cervical vaginal cytology (Bethesda Committee, 1993). In 1992, it was estimated that 87% of laboratories used the Bethesda system as measured by the College of American Pathologists 1991 Interlaboratory Comparison Program (Davey et al., 1992). The Bethesda system is also used in other nations, such as France (Cochand-Priollet and Vacher-Lavenu, in press). Diagnostic standardization allows clinicians to feel more certain that a diagnosis has the same meaning regardless of the laboratory making that diagnosis.

Interobserver diagnostic variability studies theoretically improve patient outcomes by improving the ability of pathologists to effectively use the optimal diagnostic criteria. The effect of interobserver variability on other aspects of patient care also has been examined. In an interobserver diagnostic variability study of mucinous tumors of the ovary, Raab et al. (1997b) showed that interobserver diagnostic variability may be sufficiently high to outweigh the effects of limited sampling. This means that regardless of the number of sections taken, the "errors" caused by limited sampling are similar to the differences due to interobserver diagnostic variability alone. This indicates that extensive sectioning protocols (e.g., one section per centimeter of tumor) may not actually affect ovarian mucinous tumor diagnosis (Raab et al., 1997b). This study shows how interobserver diagnostic variability affects the overall cost of diagnosis and patient prognosis.

EFFECT OF ERROR ON PATIENT OUTCOMES

True anatomic pathology errors are important to monitor because they affect the overall quality of care (Foucar, 1997, 1998; Nakleh and Zarbo, 1998; Frable, 1997; Krieger, 1997; Hocking et al., 1997; Safrin and Bark, 1993; Goldstein, in press). The two major types of anatomic pathology error are interpretive and reporting (Goldstein, in press). Interpretive errors occur during specimen grossing, intraoperative consultation, specimen handling, and microscopic evaluation. The distinction between discrepancies resulting from interpretive error and discrepancies resulting from interobserver diagnostic variability may be difficult to determine (Raab et al., 1994a), although it is generally agreed upon that cases of interpretive error occur. Reporting errors are mistakes in the anatomic pathology report (e.g., mislabeled site from where the specimen was obtained or wrong patient identification) (Goldstein, in press).

The proportion of minor diagnostic or reporting errors that have no impact on patient care has been estimated to range from 2% to 3% (Abt et al., 1995; Ramsay and Gallagher, 1992). Depending on the study materials and methods, the proportion of potentially significant diagnostic errors per pathologist ranges from 0.25% to 3.9% (Cree et al., 1993; Ramsay and Gallagher, 1992; Macartney et al., 1981; Whitehead et al., 1984, 1986). Epstein et al. found that 1.2% of all prostate needle biopsies being reviewed prior to surgery were incorrectly diagnosed as adenocarcinoma (Epstein et al., 1996). Furness and Lauder (1997) estimated that the average private practice pathologist becomes aware of one major mistake every year. Knowing anatomic pathology error rates may improve laboratory performance.

In order to decrease and determine the impact of anatomic pathology errors, audit systems have been implemented (Goldstein, in press; Ramsay and Gallagher, 1992). One type of audit system selects cases that have the potential to significantly alter patient care, whereas the other system is a random review of a percentage of all cases, regardless of the potential impact of a misdiagnosis (Goldstein, in press). Internal audit systems may take place before a case is finaled; after a case is finaled but before or during a weekly or monthly conference such as a tumor board; or during specified quarterly, semiannual, or annual sessions. Ramsey and Gallagher (1992) described an audit system in which 2% of randomly chosen cases per month were evaluated on the basis of nine parameters (including macroscopic description, reporting delays, turnaround time, and accuracy of coding).

In cytology, audits are performed for all types of specimens. The Clinical Laboratory Improvement Amendments of 1988 (CLIA '88) mandated that at least 10% of all negative cervical vaginal smears be reviewed by a second cytotechnologist before the case is finaled (CLIA '88, 1992). For patients who have a noncorrelating cytology and surgical pathology diagnosis, review of both specimen types by a pathologist is necessary (Council on Scientific Affairs, 1989; Forum, 1992; Schmidt et al., 1992). For women who are newly diagnosed with a high-grade squamous intraepithelial lesion on a Pap smear and have no history of cervical precursor lesions, retrospective review of the negative Pap smears from the previous 5 years is necessary. A major drawback in performing audits is the added cost; Safrin and Bark (1993) estimated that the cost per case for a second pathologist to review every case was approximately $7. Rescreening cervical vaginal smears has been shown to be cost-effective in select patient populations (e.g., patients with a prior history of cervical dysplasia) (Raab et al., 1999b). Rescreening has other values than detecting errors, such as improving cytotechnologist performance by providing continuous feedback (Krieger, 1997; Krieger et al., 1998).

One area in surgical pathology that has been extensively evaluated in terms of error management is the frozen section consultation. The range of overall accuracy of frozen section diagnosis is 95% to 99% (Goldstein, in press; Zarbo et al., 1991; Sherwood and Hunt, 1984; Torp and Skjorten, 1990; Dankwa and Davies, 1985; Howanitz et al.,1990; Rogers et al., 1987). Zarbo et al. (1991) estimated that in 48% of discordant cases, the discordance was due to tissue sampling. Howanitz et al. (1990) reported that a discordant frozen section diagnosis greatly affected patient management in 6% of cases. These data aid pathologists by showing the areas in which mistakes are likely to occur. These data also aid clinicians by showing that errors, although infrequent, occur in intraoperative consultations and that clinicians should always integrate frozen section diagnoses with clinical impressions (Goldstein, in press).

QUALITY IMPROVEMENT

Monitoring surgical pathology and cytology error is an example of monitoring laboratory quality (Zarbo, in press). Quality improvement guidelines have been published by a number of organizations, such as the College of American Pathologists (CAP) and the Association of Directors of Anatomic and Surgical Pathology (Zarbo, in press; Bachner et al., 1994; CPT 95, 1995; Commission on Laboratory Accreditation, CAP, 1997; JCAHO, 1997; Travers, 1993; Solomon, 1989). Quality issues may be divided into quality assurance issues, which deal with outcomes (in anatomic pathology this usually means the report), and quality control issues, which evaluate the uniformity of processes (Zarbo, in press). For example, quality control includes monitoring the quality of sectioning, staining, and mounting sections; technical and policy manuals are created to describe the ways specimens should be handled. Different organizations, such as the CAP and the American Society of Cytopathology, will inspect and accredit laboratories based on the laboratories' ability to follow specific guidelines (Zarbo, in press; Bachner et al., 1994; CPT 95, 1995; CAP, 1997; JCAHO, 1997). Quality monitors in the cytology laboratory include recording the number of slides screened by each cytotechnologist per day, using laboratory reports that distinguish specimens that are unsatisfactory for diagnostic interpretation, making sure that all atypical, premalignant, or malignant cases are referred to the pathologist (hierarchical review) for final diagnosis, and performing descriptive laboratory statistics (Zarbo, in press; Bachner et al., 1994; CPT 95, 1995; CAP, 1997; JCAHO, 1997, Travers, 1993; Solomon, 1989).

The traditional focus on quality improvement has been on the diagnosis. There is now a greater emphasis on other aspects, such as timeliness, convenience, utilization of resources, and accessibility (Travers, 1993). Performance measurement is one of the more recent accreditation-related quality initiatives. Various approaches are being used by accrediting agencies. These include the ORYX initiative by the Joint Commission of Accreditation of Healthcare Organizations, the HEDIS under the National Committee for Quality Assurance, and the Q-T'RACKS continuous performance measurement program under the College of American Pathologists (Zarbo, in press). Since 1989, anatomic pathology laboratory performance and practice benchmarking has been accomplished through the College of American Pathologists Q-Probes voluntary subscription quality improvement program (Zarbo, in press; Travers, 1993; Schifman et al., 1996; Berman et al., 1990). Over 3000 laboratories have participated since the program's inception (Zarbo, in press).

Two areas in pathology that have affected the measure of quality are the widespread use of new pathology technologies (such as flow cytometry, new cytology technologies, telepathology, immunohistochemistry, image analysis, and molecular diagnostic techniques) and medical legal issues (Travers, 1993; Berman et al., 1990; Linton and Peachey, 1990; Hilborne and Nathan, 1991; Taylor, 1992; Bosman et al., 1992). For example, the use of new cytology technologies is currently being evaluated in the medical literature and at scientific meetings (Linder, 1992; Raab et al., 1999a; Brown and Garber, 1999). New cytology technologies include automation, which may be used for primary or secondary screening, and monolayer methods, which replace the conventional cytology "smear" (Raab et al., 1999a; Brown and Garber, 1999). In order to be used in the United States, these technologies must go through a process to get federal Food and Drug Administration approval. The Intersociety Working Group of New Cytology Technologies has recommended guidelines for how these technologies should be evaluated (Bedrossian et al., 1997, 1998). In the literature, several studies have examined the cost -effectiveness of these new technologies (Raab et al., 1999a; Brown and Garber, 1999), although additional studies are needed and are being performed to evaluate other benefits of these technologies.

Diagnostic immunohistochemistry has been used for the past 20 years, and the general impression is that this technique is helpful for pathologic interpretation and clinical management (Wick et al., in press). Wick has reported that the areas where diagnostic immunohistochemistry positively affects patient outcomes are in the rapid identification of infectious organisms, the delineation of hematolymphoid cell lineage in cases of undifferentiated malignant neoplasia, and the identification of microscopic "floaters" (Wick et al., in press). Immunohistochemistry increasingly is being used to predict patient response to treatment and prognosis (Wick et al., in press). There is confusion among physicians regarding the difference between prognostic and predictive markers. Predictive markers are aimed at forecasting clinical response to a specific therapeutic approach (e.g., estrogen and progesterone receptors) (Makris et al., 1997; Yang et al., 1999). Prognostic markers are aimed at predicting patient survival. Overviews of the use of prognostic immunohistochemical markers in specific clinical situations have been reported (Wick et al., in press; Wick, 1992; Funke and Shraut, 1998; Mathieu et al., 1990; Frew et al., 1986; de Mascarel et al., 1992; Glickman et al., 1999).

Medical legal issues in anatomic pathology have centered on quality and patient outcomes (Travers, 1993). Currently there is perceived to be an adverse medical legal environment in the United States surrounding cytology laboratories. This is partly due to unrealistic expectations for cytology laboratory performance and confusion regarding the standard of practice. The medical legal climate in cervical vaginal cytology has profound implications on the quality of care of women (Austin and McLendon, 1997a, 1997b; Dugan, 1994; Godfrey, 1999; Skoumal and Cohen, 1997). The Pap smear has proved to be remarkably effective in decreasing the incidence of cervical vaginal cancer (Brown and Garber, 1999). Researchers argue that the risk of developing cervical cancer is extremely low in women who receive regular examinations and that those women who develop cancer are almost invariably women who have not had a regular Pap smear (Brown and Garber, 1999). However, the fear of lawsuits, increasing governmental regulation, low reimbursements, and increased laboratory cost of using new technologies has resulted in some pathologists opting not to examine cervical vaginal smears.

PATIENT SATISFACTION AND PREFERENCE

In many areas of medicine, patients increasingly want to play a greater role in the decision making process. Considerations of patient satisfaction and preference are important in diagnostic testing (Fottler et al., 1997; Llewel-lyn-Thomas, 1997; Cher et al., 1997). Many times there are different testing strategies, all with their own unique limitations and benefits, that may be used in the diagnostic workup (Llewellyn-Thomas, 1997). In a theoretical analysis, Raab and Hornberger (1997c) showed that patient risk aversion affected the cost-effectiveness of pulmonary diagnostic workup strategies. Workup strategies using technologies with high sensitivities (e.g., thoracoscopy) were more cost-effective in patients who were risk averse to false negative diagnoses. Workup strategies using technologies with low morbidities and mortalities (e.g., sputum cytology) were more cost-effective in patients who were risk averse to procedures with higher complication rates. These data indicate that there may not be an optimal testing strategy for all patients, and that strategies must be tailored to meet specific patient desires.

Measuring patient perceptions regarding diagnostic testing also is important in other areas, such as cervical vaginal screening and breast disease diagnosis. The anatomic pathologist plays a critical role in determining the optimal test, because he or she often has the most knowledge regarding how a diagnosis actually is made (i.e., the pathologist often knows the most about test accuracy and the nuances of establishing a diagnosis). In some areas, the pathologist actually performs the diagnostic test (e.g., breast FNA) and thus has a bias for wanting this test to be performed in lieu of other testing strategies.

COST ANALYSES

As efforts persist to provide quality care at an affordable cost, cost analysis has become a dominant issue for deciding optimal medical practice (Detsky and Naglie, 1990; Siegel et al., 1996; Roper et al., 1988), including pathology practice. Determining costs of production has been performed in some anatomic pathology areas. These costs include personnel, supplies and equipment, and overhead. For example, the cost of cytology laboratory production in cervical vaginal cytology has been determined by both Bishop (1997) and Raab et al. (1999a). These studies estimated that the cost per Pap smear for a cytology laboratory is approximately $15 (Raab et al., 1999a). The cost to process surgical pathology specimens also has been estimated. The data derived from these types of analyses may then be used in cost analyses that compare two or more types of tests or diagnostic procedures. Finkler (1982) has elucidated why it is important to separate costs from charges in medical research, and this also is true for anatomic pathology research.

The types of cost analysis that are commonly used in the medical literature include cost minimization, cost consequence, cost-effectiveness, and cost benefit analysis (Detsky and Naglie, 1990; Siegel et al., 1996; Roper et al., 1988; Bishop, 1997; Finkler, 1982; Luce et al., 1996). Although all these types of analysis measure costs, they measure the utilities or effectiveness of tests or procedures in different metrics. In cost minimization analysis the effectiveness of different tests are assumed to be equal. In cost consequence analysis, the costs and consequences of different tests are calculated separately and not combined. In cost-effectiveness analysis, costs and other outcomes are measured in the same metric across all alternatives. Cost utility analysis is a special type of cost-effectiveness analysis in which the outcomes other than costs are expressed in terms of values or utilities. This method requires that patient desires or preferences be measured and is more difficult to perform than cost-effectiveness analysis. In cost benefit analysis, all outcomes are expressed in terms of cost. This method is much more common in economics than in health care. A difficulty with this method is that monetary values must be placed on all variables including human life, and this is not always intuitive. An advantage of this type of analysis is that tests or programs may be compared across a variety of social concerns.

Cost minimization and cost-effectiveness analysis have been performed for anatomic pathology services. Using cost minimization analysis, Grzybicki et al. (in press) showed that the use of pathologists' assistants was highly beneficial. Cost-effectiveness analysis has been used to examine the utility of the histologic examination of routine tissues, cervical vaginal screening and rescreening, workup strategies in patients with lung or breast lesions, and new cytology technologies (Layfield et al., 1993; Grzybicki et al., in press; Raab, 1998; Raab et al., 1998b, 1998c, 1999a).

Cost-effectiveness analyses often incorporate a large number of variables through analytic techniques such as decision analysis, which is a normative method to summarize existing probabilistic data. Other types of studies, such as a randomized clinical trial, have rarely been performed in pathology laboratories or on the use of pathology tests.

In 1993, the U.S. Public Health Service appointed a panel of 13 health researchers and academics to review the state of the science of cost-effectiveness analyses and foster consensus to standardize the conduct of cost-effectiveness studies. The panel specified that cost-effectiveness studies should conform to specific standards, which are: (1) a statement of perspective, (2) a description of benefits, (3) a description of costs, (4) the appropriate use of discounting, (5) the use of sensitivity analysis, and (6) a report of summary measures (Siegel et al., 1996; Luce et al., 1996; Grzybicki et al., in press; Raab, 1998; Raab et al., 1998b, 1998c; Weinstein et al., 1996). In a 1992 review, Udvarhelyi et al. reported that only 3 of 77 articles conformed to all six standards. Recent pathology cost-effectiveness studies, such as the study by Brown and Garber on the cost-effectiveness of new cytology technologies, have conformed to these standards (Brown and Garber, 1999).

SUMMARY

Anatomic pathology is playing an increasingly important role in patient outcomes management. The information generated in anatomic pathology is being integrated with databases from other sources in order to improve patient care. Much of patient-centered outcomes research will be guided by anatomic pathologists as health-care providers recognize the value and meaning of anatomic pathology diagnoses.

REFERENCES

Abt AB, Abt LG, Olt GJ. The effect of interinstitution anatomic pathology consultation on patient care. *Arch. Pathol. Lab. Med.* 1995;119:514–517.

Austin RM, MeLendon WW. College of American Pathologists Conference XXX: Quality and liability issues with the Papanicolaou smear. *Arch. Pathol. Lab. Med.* l997a;121:205–342.

Austin RM. McLendon WW. Medicine's most successful cancer screening procedure is threatened. *JAMA* 1997b;277:754–755.

Bachner P, Howanitz PS, Lent RW. Quality improvement practices.in clinical and anatomic pathology services. A College of American Pathologists Q-Probes Study of the program characteristics and performance in 580 institutions. *Am. J. Clin. Pathol.* 1994;102:567–571.

Beck JR, Shultz EK. The use of relative operative characteristic (ROC) curves in test performance evaluation. *Arch. Pathol. Lab. Med.* 1986; 110:13–20.

Bedrossian C, Bonfiglio T, Coble D, Davey D, Hutchinson M, Kaufman E. Krieger P. Mody D, Raab S, Ramzv I, Rosenthal D, Saigo P. Schumann I, Solomon D, Sornrak T, Zaleski S. Proposed guidelines for primary screening instruments for gynecologic cytology. *Am. J. Clin. Pathol.* 1998a:10–15.

Bedrossian C, Bonfigilo T, Coble D, Davey O, Hutchinson M, Kaufman E, Krieger P, Mody D, Raab S, Ramzv I, Rosenthal O, Saigo P, Schumann J, Solomon ID, Somrak T, Zaleski S. Proposed guidelines for secondary screening (rescreening instruments for gynecologic cytology). *Acta Cytol.* 1998b;42:1311–1314.

Berenson RA. Capitation and conflict of interest. *Health Affairs* 1986;5:141–146.

Berman GD, Kottke TE, Ballard DJ. Effectiveness research and assessment of clinical outcome: A review of federal government and medical community involvement. *Mayo Clin. Proc.* 1990;65:657–663.

Bethesda Committee: The Bethesda systemfor reporting cervical/vaginal cytologic diagnoses. *Acta Cytol.* 1993;37:115–124.

Bishop SW. The costof production in cervical cytology: comparison of conventional and automated primary screening systems. *Am. J. Clin. Pathol.* 1997;107: 445–450.

Boerner S, Sneige N. Specimen adequacy and false-negative diagnosis rate in fine-needle aspirates of palpable breast masses. *Cancer* 1998;84:344–348.

Boerner S, Fornage BD, Singletary E, Sneige N. Ultrasound-guided fine-needle aspiration (ENA) of nonpalpable breast lesions: A review of 1885 FNA cases using the National Cancer Institute-supported recommendations on the uniform approach to breast FNA. *Cancer* 1999;87:19–24.

Bosman PT. de Goeij AFPM, Rousch M. Quality control in immunocytochemistry: Experiences with the estrogen receptor assay. *J. Clin. Pathol.* 1992;45:120–124.

Brown AD, Garber AM. Cost-effectiveness of 3 methods to enhance the sensitivity of Papanicolaou testing. *JAMA* 1999;281:347–353.

Burton EC, Troxclair DA. Newman WP III. Autopsy diagnoses of malignant neo-plasms: How often are clinical diagnoses incorrect? *JAMA* 1998;280: 1245–1248.

Cher DJ, Miyamoto S, Lenert LA. Incorporating risk attitude into Markov-process decision models: importance for individual decision making. *Med. Decision Making* 1997;17:340–350.

Clinical Laboratory Improvement Amendments of 1988. Final Rule (42 CFR Part 405, et al.). *Fed. Reg.* l992;57:7001–7186. (Also see 1993 Technical Corrections.)

Cochand-Priollet B, Vacher-Lavenu MC. French gynecological cytology. *Clin. Lab. Med.* (in press).

Cohen MB, Rodgers RPC, Hales MS, et al. Influence of training and experience in fine-needle aspiration biopsy of breast. *Arch. Pathol. Lab. Med.* 1987;111: 518–520.

Commission on Laboratory Accreditation. Inspection Checklist: Autopsy Pathology. College of American Pathologists, Northfield, IL, 1997.

Confortini M, Biggeri A, Cariaggi MlP, et al. Intralaboratory reproducibility in cervical cytology. Results of the application of a 100-slide set. *Acta Cytol.* 1993; 37:49–54.

Cooncy PE. Proposed restrictions on physician referrals to clinical labs: Important areas left unclarified. *Healthspan* 1992;9:3–7.

Council on Scientific Affairs: Quality assurance in cervical cytology. The Papanico-laou smear. *JAMA* 1989;262:1672–1679.

Cox FT. ASCP practice guidelines: management of glandular abnormalities in the cervical smear. *J. Lower Genital Tract Dis.* l997;1:41–45.

CPT 95. *Physicians' current procedural terminology.* American Medical Association, Chicago, 1995.

Cree LA, Guthrie W. Anderson SM, et al. Departmental audit in histopathology. *Pathol. Res. Pract.* 1993;189:453–457.

Dalton LW. Page DL, Dupont WD. Histologic grading of breast carcinoma. A repro-ducibility study. *Cancer* 1994;73: 2765–2770.

Dankwa EK, Davies ID. Frozen section diagnosis: An audit. *J. Clin. Pathol.* 1985;38: 1235–1240.

Davey OD, Nielsen ML, Rosenstock W, Kline TS. Terminology and specimen ade-quacy in cervicovaginal cytology. The College of American Pathologists Inter-laboratory Comparison Program experience. *Arch. Pathol. Lab. Med.* 1992;116: 903–907.

de Mascarel I, Bonichon F, Coindre JM, Trojani M. Prognostic significance of breast cancer axillary lymph node micrometastases assessed by two special techniques: Re-evaluation with longer follow-up. *Br. J. Cancer* 1992;66:523–527.

dePangher Manzini V, Revignas MG, Brollo A. Diagnosis of malignant tumor: Com-parison between clinical and autopsy diagnoses. *Hum. Pathol.* 1995;26:280–283.

Detsky AS, Naglie IG. A clinician's guide to cost-effectiveness analysis. *Ann. Intern. Med.* 1990;113:147–154.

Dugan SFX. Legal implications for the physician in the wake of automation: Medical malpractice. In: Grohs H, Husain QAN (eds.), *Automated Cervical Cancer Screening.* Igaku-Shoin, Tokyo, 1994.

Eisenburg SM, Myers LP, Pauly MV. How will changes in physician payment by Medicare influence laboratory testing? *JAMA* 1987;258:803–808.

Ellis IO, Pinder SE. Fine needle aspiration (ENA) cytology of breast: Refining the diagnosis. *Cytopathology* 1998;9:289–290.

Epstein AM, Krock SJ, McNeil BJ. Office laboratory tests. Perceptions of profitability. *Med. Care* 1984;22:160–166.

Epstein JI, Walsh PC, Sanfilippo F. Clinical and cost impact of second-opinion pathology. Review of prostate biopsies prior to radical prostatectomy. *Am. J. Surg. Pathol.* 1996;20:851–857.

Fechner RE. One century of mammary carcinoma in situ. What have we learned? *Am. J. Clin. Pathol.* 1993;100:654–661.

Finkler SA. The distinction between cost and charges. *Ann. Intern. Med.* 1982;96:102–109.

Fisher ER. Pathobiological considerations relating to the treatment of intraductal carcinoma (ductal carcinoma in situ) of the breast. *CA Cancer J. Clin* 1997;47:52–64.

Fisher B, Dignam I, Wolmark N, et al. Lumpectomy and radiation therapy for the treatment of intraductal breast cancer: Findings from National Surgical Adjuvant Breast and Bowel Project B-17. *J. Clin. Oncol.* 1998;16:441–452.

Forum: Legislation and regulations governing the field of cytology review and update. In: Schmidt WA (ed.). *Cytopathology Annual*, pp. 197–253. Williams & Wilkins, Baltimore, 1992.

Fottler MC, Ford RC, Bach SA. Measuring patient satisfaction in healthcare organizations: Qualitative and quantitative approaches. *Best Pract. Benchmarking Healthcare* 1997;2:227–239,

Foucar F. Do pathologists play dice? Uncertainty and early histopathological diagnosis of common malignancies. *Histopathology* 1997;31:495–502.

Foucar F. Error identification: a surgical pathology dilemma. *Am. J. Surg. Pathol.* 1998;22:1–5.

Frable WJ. Does a zero error standard exist for the Papanicolaou smear? A pathologist's perspective. *Arch. Pathol. Lab. Med.* 1997;121:301–10.

Fraire NE, McLarty JW, Greenberg SD. Changing utilization of cytopathology versus histopathology in the diagnosis of lung cancer. *Diagn. Cytopathol.* 1991;7:359–362.

Frew A, Ralfkiaer N, Ghosh AK, Gatter KC, Mason DY. Immunocytochemistry in the detection of bone marrow metastasis in patients with primary lung cancer. *Br. J Cancer* 1986;53:555–556.

Funke I, Schraut W. Meta-analysis of studies on bone marrow micrometastasis: An independent prognostic impact remains to be substantiated. *J. Clin. Oncol.* 1998;16:557–566.

Furness RN, Lauder IA. A questionnaire-based survey of errors in diagnostic histopathology throughout the United Kingdom. *J. Clin. Pathol.* 1997;50:457–460.

Giard RW, Hermans J. Interpretation of diagnostic cytology with likelihood ratios. *Arch. Pathol. Lab.Med.* 1990;114:852–854.

Glickman JN, Torres C, Wang HH, Turner JR, Shahsafaei A. Richards WG, Sugarbaker DJ, Odze RD. The prognostic significance of lymph node micrometastasis in patients with esophageal carcinoma. *Cancer* 1999;8(5):769–778

Godfrey SE. The Pap smear. Automated rescreening and negligent nondisclosure. *Am. J. Clin. Pathol.* 1999;111:14–17.

Goldstein NS. Diagnostic errors in surgical pathology. *Clin. Lab. Med.* (in press).

Grundmann E. Autopsy as clinical quality control: a study of 15,143 autopsy cases. *In Vivo* 1994;8:945–952.

Grzybicki DM, Galvis CO, Raab SS. The utility of pathologists assistants. *Am. J. Clin. Pathol.* (in press).

Hilborne LH. Nathan LE. Quality improvement in an era of cost containment. *Am. J. Clin. Pathol.* 1991:96(suppl.);56–59.

Hocking OR, Niteckis VN, Cairns BJ, et al. Departmental audit in surgical anatomical pathology. *Pathology* 1997;29:418–421.

Howanitz PJ, Hoffman GG, Zarbo RJ. The accuracy of frozen-section diagnoses in 34 hospitals. *Arch. Pathol. Lab. Med.* 1990;114:355–359.

Joint Commission on Accreditation of Healthcare Organizations. *Accreditation Manual for Hospitals.* JCAHO, Oakbrook Terrace, IL, 1997.

Karunaratne S, Benbow EW. A survey of general practitioners' views on autopsy reports. *J. Clin. Pathol.* 1997;50:548–552.

Krieger PA. Strategies for reducing Papanicolaou smear screening errors: Principles derived from data and experience with quality control. *Arch. Pathol. Lab. Med.* 1997;121:277–281.

Krieger PA, Cohen T, Naryshikin S. A practical guide to Papanicolaou smear re-screens: How many slides must be reevaluated to make a statistically valid assessment of screening performance? *Cancer* 1998;84:130–137.

Landefeld CS, Chren MM, Myers A et al. Diagnostic yield of the autopsy in a university hospital and a community hospital. *N. Engl. J. Med.* 1988;318: 1249–1254.

Langley FA, Buckley CM, Taster M. The use of ROC curves in histopathologic decision making. *Anal. Quant. Cytol.* 1985;7:167–173.

Layfield U, Chrischilles EA, Cohen MB, Bottles K. The palpable breast nodule. A cost-effectiveness analysis of alternate diagnostic approaches. *Cancer* 1993;72: 1642–1651.

Linder J. Automation in cytopathology. *Am. J. Clin. Pathol.* 1992;98:S47–S51.

Linton AL, Peachey DK. Guidelines for medical practice: I. The reasons why. *Can. Med. Assoc. J.* 1990;143:485–490.

Liu K, Layfield U, Coogan AC, et al. Diagnostic accuracy in fine-needle aspiration of soft tissue and bone lesions. Influence of clinical history and experience. *Am. J. Clin. Pathol.* 1999;111:632–640.

Llewellyn-Thomas HA. Investigating patients' preferences for different treatment options. *Can. J. Nurs. Res.* 1997;29:45–64.

Luce B, Manning W, Siegel S, Lipscomb J. Estimating costs in cost-effectiveness analysis. In: Gold M, Siegel A, Russell L, Weinstein M. (eds.). *Cost-Effectiveness in Health and Medicine*, pp. 176–213. Oxford University Press, New York, 1996.

Macartney IC, Henson DE, Codling BW. Quality assurance in anatomic pathology. *Am. J. Clin. Pathol.* 1981;7:467–475.

Makris A, Powles TJ, Dowsett M, et al. Prediction of response to neoadjuvant chemoendocrine therapy in primary breast carcinomas. *Clin. Cancer Res.* 1997;3:593–600.

Mathieu MC, Friedman S., Bosq S, Caillou B. Spielmann M, Travagli JP, Contesso G. Immunohistochemical staining of bone marrow biopsies for detection of occult metastasis in breast cancer. *Breast Cancer Res. Treat.* 1990;15:21–26.

McNeil BJ, Ranley JA. Statistical approaches to the analysis of receiver operating characteristic (ROC) curves. *Med. Decision Making* 1984; 4:137–150.

Metz CE. ROC methodology in radiologic imaging. *Invest. Radiol.* 1986;21:720–733.

Morretin IBM. Conflicts of interest. Profits and problems in physician referrals. *JAMA* 1989;262:390–394.

Nakhleh RE, Zarbo RI. Amended reports in surgical pathology and implications for diagnostic error detection and avoidance: A College of American Pathologists Q-probes study of 1,667,547 accessioned cases in 359 laboratories. *Arch. Pathol. Lab. Med.* 1998;122:303–309.

O'Sullivan JP. Observer variation in gynaecological cytopathology. *Cytopathology* 1998;9:6–14.

Oweity T, Hughes JH, Cohen MB, et al. The effect of patient history on diagnostic accuracy in the interpretation of bronchial brush specimens. *Acta Cytol.* 1998;42:1262.

Page DL, Dupont WV. Benign breast diseases and premalignant breast disease. *Arch. Pathol. Lab. Med.* 1998;122:1048–1050.

Page DL, Jensen RA, Simpson IF. Premalignant and malignant disease of the breast: The roles of the pathologist. *Mod. Pathol.* 1998;11:120–128.

Page DL, Simpson JE, Ductal carcinoma in situ—The focus for prevention, screening, and breast conservation in breast cancer. *N. Engl. J. Med.* 1999;340: 1499–1500.

Raab SS. Diagnostic accuracy in cytopathology. *Diagn. Cytopathol.* 1994;10:68–75.

Raab SS, Bottles K, Cohen MB. Technology assessment in anatomic pathology: An illustration of technology assessment techniques in fine needle aspiration biopsy. *Arch. Pathol. Lab. Med.* 1994a;181:1173–1180.

Raab SS, Lend JC, Cohen MB. Low grade transitional cell carcinoma of the bladder: Key cytomorphologic features as identified by regression analysis. *Cancer* 1994b;74:1621–1626.

Raab SS, Thomas PA, Lend JC, et al. Pathology and probability. Likelihood ratios and receiver operating characteristic curves in the interpretation of bronchial brush specimens. *Am. J. Clin. Pathol.* 1995;103:588–593.

Raab SS, Slagel DD, Jensen CS, et al. Low grade transitional cell carcinoma of the urinary bladder: Application of select cytologic criteria to improve diagnostic accuracy. *Mod. Pathol.* 1996;9:225–232.

Raab SS, Snider TE, Potts SA, et al. Atypical glandular cells of undetermined significance: Diagnostic accuracy and interobserver variability using select cytologic criteria. *Am. J. Clin. Pathol.* 1997a;107:299–307.

Raab SS, Robinson RA, Jensen CS, et al. Mucinous tumors of the ovary: Interobserver variability and utility of sectioning protocols. *Arch. Pathol. Lab. Med.* 1997b;121:1192–1198.

Raab SS, Hornberger J. The effect of a patient's risk-taking attitude on the cost effectiveness of testing strategies in the evaluation of pulmonary lesions. *Chest* 1997c;111:1583–1590.

Raab SS. The cost effectiveness of routine histologic examination. *Am. J. Clin. Pathol.* 1998;110:391–396.

Raab SS, Geisinger KR, Silverman JF, et al. Interobserver variability of a Pap smear diagnosis of atypical glandular cells of undetermined significance (AGUS). *Am. J. Clin. Pathol.* 1998a;110:653–659.

Raab SS, Slagel DD, Robinson RA. The utility of the histologic examination of tissue removed during elective joint replacement: A preliminary assessment. *J. Bone Joint Surg.* 1998b;80A:331–335.

Raab SS, Steiner AL, Hornberger S. The cost effectiveness of treating women with a cervical vaginal smear diagnosis of atypical squamous cells of undetermined significance. *Am. J. Obstet. Gynecol.* 1998c;179:411–420.

Raab SS, Zaleski MS, Silverman JF. The cost effectiveness of the cytology laboratory and new cytology technologies in cervical cancer prevention. *Am. J. Clin. Pathol.* 1999a;109:259–266.

Raab SS, Bishop NS, Zaleski MS. Cost effectiveness of rescreening cervicovaginal smears. *Am. J. Clin. Pathol.* 1999b;111:601–609.

Raab SS, Gross T, Grzybicki DM, Silverman JF. Clinical perception of the utility of sputa and other tests in patients with lung masses. *Mod. Pathol.* 1999c;12:188.

Radack KL. Rouan O, Hedges J. The likelihood ratio: An improved measure for reporting and evaluating diagnostic test results. *Arch. Pathol. Lab. Med.* 1986;110:689–693

Ramsay AD, Gallagher PJ. Local audit of surgical pathology. *Am. J. Surg. Pathol.* 1992;16:476–482.

Ranley JA, McNeil BI. The meaning and use of the area under a receiver operating characteristic (ROC) curve. *Radiology* 1982;143:29–36.

Renshaw AA, Dean BR, Cibas ES. Receiver operating characteristic curves for analysis of the results of cervicovaginal smears. A useful quality improvement tool. *Arch. Pathol. Lab. Med.* 1997;121:968–975.

Rogers C, Klatt EC, Chandrasoma P. Accuracy of frozen-section diagnosis in a teaching hospital. *Arch. Pathol. Lab. Med.* 1987;111:54–57.

Roper WL, Windenwerder W, Hackbarth GM, Krakauer H. Effectiveness in health care: an initiative to evaluate and improve medical practice. *N. Engl. J. Med.* 1988;319:1197–1202.

Rosai J. Borderline epithelial lesions of the breast. *Am. J. Surg. Pathol.* 1991;15: 209–21.

Rosen PP. Proliferative breast "disease." An unresolved diagnostic dilemma. *Cancer* 1993;71:3798–3807.

Rosen PP, Lesser ML, Arroyo CD, et al. Immunohistochemical detection of HER2-neu in patients with axillary lymph node negative breast carcinoma. A study of epidemiologic risk factors, histologic features, and prognosis. *Cancer* 1995;75:1320–1326.

Ross JS, Fletcher JA. The HER-2/neu oncogene in breast cancer: Prognostic factor, predictive factor, and target for therapy. *Stem Cells* 1998;16:413–428.

Sackett DL, Haynes RB, Guyatt GM, Tugwell P. *Clinical Epidemiology: A Basic Science for Clinical Medicine*, second edition. Little, Brown, Boston, 1991.

Safrin RE, Bark CI. Surgical pathology sign-out. Routine review of every case by a second pathologist. *Am. J. Surg. Pathol.* 1993,17:1190–1192.

Sanchez MA, Stahl RE. Fine-needle aspiration of the breast. *Pathology (Phila.)*1996;4:253–286.

Santoso IT, Colernan RL, Voet RL. Pathology slide review in gynecologic oncology. *Obstet. Gynecol.* 1998;91:730–734.

Sarode VR, Datta BN, Banerjee AK, et al., Autopsy findings and clinical diagnoses: A review of 1,000 cases. *Hum. Pathol.* 1993;24:194–198.

Schifman RB, Howanitz PJ, Zarbo RJ. Q-probes: A College of American Pathologists benchmarking program for quality management in pathology and laboratory medicine. In: Weinstein RS (ed.), *Advances in Pathology and Laboratory Medicine*, pp. 83–120. Mosby-Yearbook, Chicago, 1996.

Schnitt SI, Connolly JL, Tavassoli PA et al. Interobserver reproducibility in the diagnosis of ductal proliferative breast lesions using standardized criteria. *Am. J. Surg. Pathol.* 1992;16:1133–1143.

Schnitt SJ. Microinvasive carcinoma of the breast: A diagnosis in search of a definition. *Adv. Anat. Pathol.* 1998;5:367–372.

Schroeder SA, Showstack JA. Financial incentives to perform medical procedures and laboratory tests: Illustrative models of office practice. *Med. Care* 1978;16: 289–298.

Schwartz WB, Wolfe RJ, Panker SO. Pathology and probabilities: A new approach to interpreting and reporting biopsies. *N. Engl. J. Med.* 1981;305:917–923.

Scott MA, Lagios MD, Axelsson K, et al. Ductal carcinoma in situ of the breast: Reproducibility of histological subtype analysis. *Hum. Pathol.* 1997;28:967–73.

Sherman ME, Schiffman MH, Erozan YS et al. The Bethesda System. A proposal for reporting abnormal cervical smears based on the reproducibility of cytopathologic diagnoses. *Arch. Pathol. Lab. Med.* 1992;116:1155–1158.

Sherman ME, Schiffman MU, Lorincz AT, et al. Toward objective quality assurance in cervical cytopathology. Correlation of cytopathologic diagnoses with detection of high-risk human papillomavirus types. *Am. J. Clin. Pathol.* 1994;102: 182–187.

Sherwood AS, Hunt AC. An external quality assessment scheme in histopathology. *J. Clin. Pathol.* 1984;37:414.

Siegel J, Weinstein M, Torrance G. Reporting cost-effectiveness studies and results. In: Gold M, Siegel J, Russell L, Weinstein M (eds.). *Cost-Effectiveness in Health and Medicine,* pp. 276–303. Oxford University Press, New York, 1996.

Silverberg SO. The institutional pathology consultation. Documentation of its importance in patient management. *Arch. Pathol. Lab. Med.* 1995;119:493.

Skoumal SM. Cohen MB. Automated cytologic screening devices and malpractice liability. *Diagn. Cytopathol.* 1997;17:85–87.

Snead DR, Vryenhoef P, Pinder SE, et al., Routine audit of breast fine needle aspiration (FNA) cytology specimens and aspirator inadequate rates. *Cytopathology* 1997;8:236–247.

Solomon B. Introduction to the proceedings of the conference on the state of the art in quality control measures for diagnostic cytology laboratories. *Acta Cytol.* 1989;319:427–430.

Steffee CR, Segletes LA, Geisinger KR. Changing cytologic and histologic utilization patterns in the diagnosis of 515 primary lung malignancies. *Cancer Cytopathol.* 1997;81:105–115.

Stevanovic O, Tucakovic O, Doflic R, et al. Correlation of clinical diagnoses with autopsy findings: A retrospective study of 2,145 consecutive autopsies. *Hum. Pathol.* 1986;17:1225–1230.

Szende B, Kendrey O, Lapis K, et al. Accuracy of admission and clinical diagnosis of tumours as revealed by 2000 autopsies. *Eur. J. Cancer* 1996;32A:1102–1108.

Taylor CR. Quality improvement and standardization in immunohistochemistry. A proposal for the annual meeting of the Biological Stain Commission. June 1991. *Biotechnol. Histochem.* 1992;67;110–117.

Toogood JR. What do we mean by "usually"? *Lancet* 1980;1:1094

Torp SH, Skjorten FJ. The reliability of frozen section diagnosis. *Acta Chir. Scand.* 1990;156:127–130.

Travers H. *Quality Improvement. Manual in Anatomic Pathology.* College of American Pathologists, Northfield, IL, 1993.

Udvarhelyi IS, Colditz GA, Pai A, Epstein AM. Cost-effectiveness and cost-benefit analyses in the medical literature. *Ann. Intern. Med.* 1992;116:238–244.

Veress B, Alafuzoff I. Clinical diagnostic accuracy audited by autopsy in a university hospital in two eras. *Qual. Assur. Health Care* 1993;5:281–286.

Veress B, Alafuzoff I. A retrospective analysis of clinical diagnoses and autopsy findings in 3,042 cases during two different time periods. *Hum. Pathol.* 1994;25:140–145.

Weinstein MC, Siegel JE, Gold MR, et al. Recommendations of the panel on cost effectiveness in health and medicine. *JAMA* 1996;276:1253–1258.

Whitehead ME, Fitzwater JE, Lindsay SK, et al. Quality assurance of histopathologic diagnoses: A prospective audit of three thousand cases. *Am. J. Clin. Pathol.* 1984;81:487–491.

Whitehead ME, Grieve JHK, Payne MJ. Quality assurance of histopathologic diagnosis in the British Army: Role of the Army Histopathologic Registry in completed case review. *J. R. Army Med. Corps* 1986;132:71–75.

Wick MR. Oncogene analysis in diagnostic pathology: A current perspective. *Am. J. Clin. Pathol.* 1992:97(suppl.):S1–S3.

Wick MR, Ritter Ml, Swanson PE. The impact of diagnostic immunohistochemistry on patient outcomes. *Clin. Lab. Med.* (in press)

Yang X, Uziely B, Groshen S, et al. MDR1 gene expression in primary and advanced breast cancer. *Lab. Invest.* 1999;79:271–280.

Yobs AR, Plott NE, Hicklin MD. Retrospective evaluation of gynecologic cytodiagnosis. II. Interlaboratory reproducibility as shown in rescreening large consecutive samples of reported cases. *Acta Cytol.* 1987;31:900–910.

Young NA, Naryshicin S, Atkinson BF et al. Interobserver variability of cervical smears with squamous-cell abnormalities: A Philadelphia study. *Diagn. Cytopathol.* 1994;11:352–357.

Zarbo RJ, Hoffman GO, Howanitz PS. Interinstitutional comparison of frozen section consultation. *Arch. Pathol. Lab. Med.* 1991;115:1187–1194.

Zarbo RJ. Monitoring anatomic pathology practice through quality assurance monitors. *Clin. Lab. Med.* (in press).

Index

Laboratory information
  for decision support, 91–92
  useful, data conversion to, 92–93
  value of, 6, 11–14
Laboratory information systems, 71
Laboratory outcomes
  applications of, 8–9
  conceptual basics of, 6–9
  for decision support, 91–126
  economic background of, 5–6
  first-order, 7
  historical background of, 3–5
  linear regression models of, 95, 101,
    123
  logistic regression models of, 95, 101, 113,
    123
  log-linear models of, 95
  multiple regression model of, 101
  second-order, 7
  third-order, 7
Laboratory outcomes research, 147–148
  challenge of study design for, 92
  components of, 93
  data analysis methods for, 101–104
  funding for, 18
  initiatives in, 15–22
  national model for
    development of, 20–21
    lack of, 20
  problems with, 16
  real-time access to, 8
  statistical analysis of, 8
  statistical framework for, 93–95
  structured data matrix for, 93
Laboratory services
  access to, 11–13
  accuracy of, 18–19
  analytical precision of, 18–19
  clinical, 129–130
  costs of, 11–12
    versus outcome, 5–6
  health services research perspective of,
    11–14
  impact on disease incidence and preva-
    lence, 4–5
  medical necessity of, 12–13
  performance indicators for, 18
  point-of-care, assessment of, 19
  in primary care, problems with, 17–18
  proficiency testing of, 147
  quality of, 11–13
    definition of, 6
    determination of, 6
  regulation of, 12–13

value of, conceptual framework for assessment, 13–14
Laboratory tests
  accuracy of, 147–160
  in ambulatory setting, 129–146
  for case-finding, 129–146
    evaluation of, 135–141
    issues in, 141–144
    predictive value of, 132
    U.S. Preventive Services Task Force rec-
      ommendations for, 140–141
  cost-effectiveness of, 164
  cycle, problems in, 141–143
  definitions, 130–132
  diagnostic, 130. *See also* Anatomic pathol-
    ogy
    patient satisfaction and preference in,
      170–171
  effectiveness of, 133, 136
    definition of, 131–132
    need for evidence, 141
  efficacy of, 133
    definition of, 131–132
  evaluation of, conceptual framework for,
    133–134
  general population versus selected popula-
    tion, 130–131
  genetic, 143–144
  in hospital setting, 130
  for monitoring, 130
  monitoring of, 130
    classification and regression tree analy-
      sis for, 155
    cost-effectiveness of, 156–157
    data-mining approach for, 155–156
    downstream event, 17, 147–160
    and patient outcomes, 147–160
    split-sample testing for, 156
  most common, 92
  multiphasic, 136
  ordering
    financial incentives for, 129
    inappropriate, 141
    indications for, 130
    preferential, 164
  and patient management, 133–134
  and patient outcomes, 133–134, 147–160
  performance characteristics of, 133
preoperative, 134–135
  goal of, 134
  Mayo Clinic guidelines for, 134–135
  for prognosis, 130
  for screening, 129–146
  yield of, 133–140